中医的理性

The Reasoning
of Traditional
Chinese Medicine

中医的理性

The Reasoning
of Traditional
Chinese Medicine

Professor **Song Xuan Ke**
Asanté Academy, UK

柯松轩教授

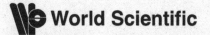

World Scientific

NEW JERSEY · LONDON · SINGAPORE · BEIJING · SHANGHAI · HONG KONG · TAIPEI · CHENNAI · TOKYO

Published by

World Scientific Publishing Europe Ltd.

57 Shelton Street, Covent Garden, London WC2H 9HE

Head office: 5 Toh Tuck Link, Singapore 596224

USA office: 27 Warren Street, Suite 401-402, Hackensack, NJ 07601

Library of Congress Cataloging-in-Publication Data

Names: Ke, Song Xuan, author.

Title: The reasoning of traditional Chinese medicine / Professor Song Xuan Ke, Asanté Academy, UK.

Description: New Jersey: World Scientific, [2023] | Includes bibliographical references and index.

Identifiers: LCCN 2022036156 | ISBN 9781800613072 (hardcover) |
    ISBN 9781800613171 (paperback) | ISBN 9781800613089 (ebook) |
    ISBN 9781800613096 (ebook other)

Subjects: LCSH: Medicine, Chinese.

Classification: LCC R601 .K47 2023 | DDC 610/.951--dc23/eng/20220727

LC record available at https://lccn.loc.gov/2022036156

British Library Cataloguing-in-Publication Data

A catalogue record for this book is available from the British Library.

For any available supplementary material, please visit
https://www.worldscientific.com/worldscibooks/10.1142/Q0386#t=suppl

Desk Editors: Sanjay Varadharajan/Adam Binnie/Shi Ying Koe

Typeset by Stallion Press
Email: enquiries@stallionpress.com

I would like to dedicate this book to my late father Zheng Dong Ke, who persuaded me to study TCM when I was a child. After over 40 years of this journey, I still enjoy it.

Preface

Humans mimic Heaven and Earth; they are matched with Sun and Moon.

Yellow Emperor's Canon of Medicine
(*Huang Di Nei Jing*), chapter 'Ling Su'

I have been practicing and teaching Traditional Chinese Medicine (TCM) for over 50 years: first in my native China and since 1987 across the United Kingdom. When I see patients in China, I will use TCM terminology, such as Heat, Cold, and Dampness. Although not every Chinese patient will fully understand the meaning of every term, a cultural continuity ensures they will at least follow the gist. Understanding the logic helps in understanding a treatment plan; and through such understanding, I have found patients more active in following the advice I give on lifestyle, diet, and behaviour.

For my Western patients, the scenario is quite different. If I explain that there is excessive Heat, Cold, or

Dampness in a patient, they will not instinctively understand what I mean, and he or she may struggle to accept the diagnosis that follows.[1] Some might then tell their Western doctor of this diagnosis, with much lost in translation, and — misunderstanding the full meaning — will illicit dismissive replies.[2]

Observing this dynamic, I have come to recognise a fundamental breakdown of communication between Chinese doctors, Western patients, and Western medicine. Superficial language differences aside, there exist deep gulfs between Eastern and Western cultures that in turn lead to substantial misunderstandings. In this era of globalisation, I believe much potential for collaboration is squandered by these misunderstandings, and it is the bridging of such gulfs that this book seeks to extend.

I began my studies of TCM at the age of 13 when as an apprentice I would collect wild herbs in the mountains and lakes of Hubei. In my later teens, I learned from local specialists how to cultivate and harvest farm-grown herbs, and when old enough, I went on to study Traditional Chinese Medicine at Guangzhou

---

[1] Especially if their temperature is normal and their skin is not damp — to the Western mind, it would make sense to reject such a diagnosis! Not understanding the significance of these terms in a TCM context.

[2] In such cases, I never blame the doctor: If a message is passed on without full understanding, it may be quite reasonable to dismiss it; were I in the Western doctor's shoes, I would no doubt do the same!

University, whose faculty maintains a long and distin-
guished history as a centre of TCM learning in
Southern China. Having graduated, I moved to London
to practice as a doctor and teacher, where I have based
my principal practice ever since. Perhaps it is this contrast that has left me feeling obligated to write
this book: a sense that I might bridge the gap between
these disparate traditions — and to marry them with
mutual understanding.

Through years of practice, I have learned that introducing TCM to the Western mind first requires one to
situate the tradition in its proper background. Without
conveying the philosophical and cultural notions that
provide the foundations of TCM, all attempts at communication will lead us to dead ends. As such, this
book aims to explain what TCM is and how it works
by explaining how it sits within a broader cultural
framework.

I am not a scientist. I will not try to explain all TCM
with scientific logic, or with excessive terminology.[3]
Instead, I intend to follow the old way: exploring the
truths of TCM with its *own* logic — explaining what it
is, and how it works, in its own language. I call this the
'Reasoning of TCM'.

---

[3] Though I do lay down the gauntlet, perhaps a scientist will take
up the challenge after me!

This is not a book on medical ethics. I will not argue on the value or weakness of TCM, whether it is right or wrong, good or bad. Following the reasoning of TCM, I will instead explain how ancient Chinese thought considers health, illness, and its treatment. As one of the oldest traditions in the world, a vast collection of books, stories, and texts exist that explain TCM. And across its thousands of years of evolution, many forms of TCM exist and have existed. Considering its totality, I find myself stuck in a hole of my own making, with the task ahead perhaps too big for me. But regardless, I will persist and try my best, with the hope that I might use my many years of clinical experience and teaching knowledge to provide a simple explanation of the Tradition.

With simplicity in mind, this study will tackle only the core elements of TCM: working to avoid becoming tanged in detail. As with any practice, many minor or regional details in TCM are very much debatable. Equally, progress continues to develop in TCM as it does in any field — with new fashions arising and new discoveries becoming commonplace. To allow ourselves to become lost in these thickets would only take us further from our goal of conveying the general sense of Traditional Chinese Medicine; so, where possible, I will avoid these distractions.

Diving into a discipline full tilt, there will be concepts that at first seem confusing, especially where terminology is involved. In TCM, where much of the terminology derives from roots in ancient Chinese language, such terms are difficult enough for modern Chinese students to fully understand. Where the use of such a term is necessary, I will pause to explore its meaning and origin. However, to fully appreciate a new concept, we must first encounter it in several contexts. So, I ask the reader to bear with me and to keep their faith with this text — trusting that understanding will develop through experience and exposure.

It is my privately held belief that the many years I have spent working with TCM have benefitted me immensely — providing me with a personal path towards health, happiness, and peace. Despite — and, as we shall see, accounting *for* — my many faults, TCM has helped to make me a more balanced person.

About the Author

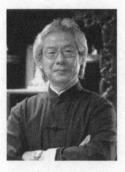 **Song Xuan Ke**, founder and principal of Asanté Academy of Chinese Medicine, has practiced and taught Traditional Chinese Medicine worldwide for over 40 years. He started to learn Chinese Medicine when he was a 13-year-old boy and an apprentice to three herbal masters in his home province of Hubei, China. He came to teach Chinese Medicine in London from 1986.

His clinical success as a leading consultant of Chinese Medicine in the UK has been featured in *The Observer*, *Daily Mail*, the *Financial Times* and on *BBC*, *CNN*, *ITV*, *Channel 4* and many other media outlets throughout the world. He is twice listed in *London Evening Standard*'s Top 50 Health Practitioners and London's 100 Best Alternative Experts, respectively. He is "simply brilliant" (quoted from *London Evening Standard* 8th May 2001).

Professor Ke has also been successfully promoting and providing acupuncture services in NHS hospitals in London and was instrumental in setting up the first BSc (Hons) and MSc courses in Chinese Medicine at a London University.

He is well known for the treatment of many chronic diseases, and he always believes that the best treatment is prevention.

Acknowledgements

I would like to thank my teachers Mr. Y. Zhao and Mr. Zhong Fa Wang back in China. I started to follow them when they went to collect wild herbs and I saw them using folk remedies to treat people, which gave me first-hand impressions and knowledge of TCM. From that, I started my journey with Chinese Medicine. I would also like to thank my university in Guangzhou for training me to become a proper TCM doctor and teacher. During the years I worked as teacher at the university, I was fortunate enough to have the opportunity to consolidate my skills and experience in teaching abroad.

I would like to express my gratitude to all who have helped me in writing this book, Christopher Ross, Rose Zhang, Alex Lusted, and of course my dear daughter Jessie. My daughter Jessie is a Western doctor and her editing, comments, and feedback on the book have been very valuable.

I also wish to express my thanks to Dr. Natalie K. Watson and Adam Binnie at World Scientific Publishing Europe for their help, guidance, and patience during the process of producing this book.

Contents

Chapter 1

An Introduction to TCM

Part One: A Brief Overview

Traditional Chinese Medicine (TCM) has been used for centuries in China, and recent decades have seen it rapidly gain popularity in the West. In turn, this development has brought new and greater scrutiny upon TCM: with its efficacy, safety, ethics, and cost-effectiveness all facing heavy critique. Above all, its scientific credentials are frequently challenged, with questions such as 'Is TCM "real medicine"?', 'What evidence supports the underlying theory and practice?', and 'How does it work in a scientific sense?', a common Western response.

For the very survival of TCM, these questions need to be answered sooner rather than later. It is undoubtedly an important task to examine the evidence and provide a fact-based explanation of TCM. However, before we commit all our energy, time, and resources to finding *scientific* justifications from the position of a

Western-medicinal framework, perhaps we might pause, consider, and ask ourselves, is this the best perspective with which to approach the truth of TCM? Does it make sense to ask questions in one language when the truth of a statement is present in another?

What do we mean by truth? Such questions imply that it is only through science that one can uncover truth. But is it the only way?

The question 'Is TCM scientific?' begs the response 'Does TCM, as a form of cultural knowledge and practice concerned with human beings, need to be purely scientific?'

Suppose, however, that we have the answer, and we decide that TCM is 'unscientific', what follows? Do we just abandon it? Perhaps we should remind ourselves that in the history of world science many notions that were at one time considered false later came to be accepted.[1] 'Science' is not fixed, and the 'truth' in science is not fixed either: rather, scientific consensus shifts over time, implying the truth behind that science is relative to whatever consensus supports it. On raw scientific principles, elements of TCM might be

---

[1] The Chinese philosopher Zhuang Zhou (c. 369–286 B.C.) wrote extensively on the nature of animal speciation, as it occurs over long periods of time, and in response to changing environmental conditions: a notion that was dismissed by Western observers until *The Origin of Species*.

rejected now, but it should not surprise us to see those judgements reversed in years to come.

TCM is a form of knowledge about the whole human being: physical and emotional, body, and mind. It has its own methodology, and this methodology is very different from that of Western scientific medicine. The way it approaches the body is different; the standards by which it judges health and illness are all different. Just as the Olympic Committee does not use football rules to referee its basketball tournament, so in the same way it is not plausible to judge one medical culture by the standards of another.

I do not dismiss the value of scientific studies into TCM. Indeed, as a society I believe we should conduct more, especially since the quality of many existing studies has been much criticised. In this book, however, I would like to take a different approach. The focus will not be on the scientific credentials of acupuncture and TCM. I will rather examine its fundamental philosophy and reasoning.

Reasoning is the basis of all knowledge, including science, and it is the application of reason that differentiates us from other animals. The search for knowledge, or truth, requires an open-minded attitude to *all* forms of reasoning: whether they be new or old, modern, or ancient, evaluating each on the basis of its own merits — under the condition of its own contexts.

In that spirit, this first chapter will deal with the question — 'What is TCM?' — which, in answering, will involve a brief exploration of its origins and history.

It should be understood throughout this discussion that although we speak of TCM, there is in practice no such thing as 'Traditional' Chinese medicine. Chinese medicine has been evolving over thousands of years, and across an exceptionally large geographical area, such that it has developed many variants, with different — and at times, competing — schools, theories, and methods. Our purpose is not to disproportionately advocate or defend any one single approach, but to address the core knowledge and common principles which can be found at the basis of TCM across all these various forms.

Part Two: What is TCM?

When discussing TCM, it is important to stress that we are not simply describing a new therapy, such as 'Gene Therapy' or 'Laser Therapy', but rather an entire medical system that stands in parallel to the 'Western' and 'Modern' medicines a British or American mind may be familiar with. The difference exists not only in the language and medical terminology used (such as 'Qi', 'Yin', and 'Yang') but more substantially in its fundamental guiding philosophical principles, contexts, and methodologies.

Traditional Chinese Medicine, which may also be called Chinese Medicine (CM), is a unique medical system which developed in China over two and half thousand years ago,[2] and now has roughly a billion adherents around the world: in and around China and other East Asian countries, including Japan, Korea, and Vietnam.

In Japan, the tradition is called 'Kampo', in Korea 'Han Yi', and in Vietnam 'Dong Yi'. While they differ in language and method, these variants all originate from historic roots in China, and therefore share the same major theories, themes, and guiding principles. What we 'are' as human beings, how our bodies function, why and how we get ill, how we might combat illness, how we can prevent illness from developing — the core concepts are universal. The essential elements are common to all forms: 'Qi'; 'Yin-Yang'; 'Jing-Qi-Shen'; and the theory of 'Five Elements': these essential elements are the common building blocks of all forms of TCM.

Equally common to all its variants are the general practices of TCM — and before exploring these terms, and the theoretical structures they contribute to, it would help us in our definition to explore what exactly these practices are.

---

[2] According to the written records, there are some texts from 2500 years ago.

Herbal Medicine Therapy

Herbal Therapy uses mainly plant-based medicines to treat illness.[3] A national guidebook on medicinal materials called *Encyclopedia of Traditional Chinese Medicine*[4] shows that nowadays in China, there are 5767 medicinal materials, which include 4773 plants,[5] 740 zoological products, and 82 minerals.

Many modern Western medicines originate from plants, e.g., aspirin from willow tree bark. However, these are no longer herbal medicines, because they are based on the extraction of certain compounds or involve the isolation and production of these compounds synthetically. These are more concentrated, more potent, and quicker acting than their herbal equivalents, but are also potentially more dangerous.

The herbal therapies in TCM are used in their original forms, such as roots, flowers, leaves, seeds, and barks, with very little processing — produced with the same

---

[3] Although occasionally animal and mineral products are used. A good deal of controversy has surrounded supposed use of animal products in TCM — and while historically there may be some truth to this — modern TCM substitutes herbal and inorganic solutions: dramatically reducing the degree and scale of use.

[4] Written by Nanjing University of Chinese Medicine and published by Shanghai Science Press (2006).

[5] This figure includes 1208 subspecies, varieties, and forms, and spans 385 families and 2313 genera.

methods used to prepare food.[6] TCM medicines in short are less concentrated, less powerful, and slower acting.

Many Chinese people have been using these forms of herbal therapy for centuries without seeing adverse side effects, so they naturally consider Chinese herbal medicines more reliable, safer, with fewer and less severe side effects. Of course, this presumption or conclusion should be challenged through scientific examination.

The most common forms of Chinese herbal medicines are teas (also known as 'decoctions'), powders, and pills: the latter of which are only loosely bound together. Western patients are often surprised when prescribed Chinese herbal therapies, as they are advised to take a large quantity: sometimes hundreds of little pills in one go. This is a consequence of this fundamental difference: with TCM, herbal pills far less concentrated in their active ingredients than the refined, synthetic Western equivalents, requiring more to achieve a similar therapeutic effect.[7]

---

[6]For example, grinding, boiling, baking, and steaming.

[7]When this logic is explained, some Western patients will ask why the pills aren't simply made in a more concentrated fashion, to reduce the total quantity. Indeed, some companies are trying to do this! But the danger follows that these patients may find it difficult to digest and absorb such products. We might have a scenario where patients have the right diagnosis and the right medicines, but in the wrong form: and they might therefore get

In addition to the difference in concentration and constitution, another key difference between traditional Chinese and Western medicines is in the way they are used. For example, a Western doctor might suggest a painkiller, or antibiotics, to address a painful tooth. In Chinese herbal medicine, however, we might consider the toothache a superficial symptom, reflecting the deeper cause, e.g., an over-accumulation of 'Heat' in the body, such that it behaves as a toxin. Therefore, a TCM doctor may suggest strong laxatives to open the patient's bowels, letting the Heat out, and diminishing the pain naturally. Why? I will return to this later — when discussing the underlying principles.

Acupuncture Therapy

Acupuncture is a set of procedures that stimulate the body's 'acupuncture points', with the intention of correcting an imbalance in the flow of 'Qi' (or 'energy') by the opening of 'channels', known as 'meridians'. Through this balance or homeostasis of Qi flow, acupuncture can promote the healing of the body.

TCM identifies 14 major meridians in the human body, between which there run many smaller channels. Along those meridians, there stand 360 acupuncture points. The idea of Qi and meridians is a unique concept, rooted in ancient Chinese tradition. The details will be

---

worse, not better. Therefore, most TCM doctors still prefer the loose forms of the medicines: as teas or herbal pills.

explained later, but briefly, this may be compared to the pattern of energy affecting the Earth. On Earth, gravity acts as a universal force, but its consequences affect different geographical points differently, according to the topography of the planet. These forces — powerful, but invisible to the eye — echo the action of Qi and meridians upon the body.

The needles used in acupuncture have changed over time, from ancient stone, bronze, iron, silver, and gold to the stainless steel used today.[8] However, the points and meridians themselves have not changed. Traditional acupuncturists consider that following the traditional acupuncture points and meridians is of key importance in treatment, while some contemporary practitioners use acupuncture without following this approach, claiming the results are just as good. This subject needs greater investigation but falls outside the scope of this book.

Tuina Therapy

Tuina is a special type of massage, which not only massages the tissues but also stimulates the acupuncture points and meridians: in a similar way to acupuncture therapy, but without needles, using only hands or feet. The purpose, as with acupuncture, is to restore balance

---

[8] Other contemporary forms include electrical, magnetic, and laser acupuncture: whatever stimulates the acupuncture sites.

where there is imbalance — a logic explored in depth in Chapter 7.

Cupping Therapy

This therapy employs 'cups', which can be made from glass, ceramics, wood, bamboo, metal, or plastic, to create local suction on the skin to draw out 'bad' Qi (energy), such as stagnated Qi, while stimulating the flow of 'good' Qi and 'Blood'.[9] It is an ancient form of therapy which belongs not only to China but also has roots in parts of Europe. The suction is affected by creating a vacuum, which can be made by briefly inserting a flame into the cup, or by withdrawing air through a device similar to a syringe.

This therapy is restricted to certain conditions and certain people. Those who are judged too fragile, too thin, too sensitive, or too elderly are advised to avoid it. It is also important to warn patients new to cupping that the process easily leaves marks on the skin (which usually disappear within a few days) and which in rare cases can cause blistering.

---

[9] In TCM, the meaning of 'Blood' is different from that in Western medicine. Partially, Blood in TCM refers to the blood as we see the red liquid flowing in the blood vessels, like Western medicine. It also refers to some other Body Waters and lymph fluids, as well as the force in the blood vessels which moves the blood.

Moxibustion Therapy

'Moxibustion' involves the combustion of a herb called Ai Ye 'moxa' (*Folium Artemisiae Argyi* — Mugwort in common English) to facilitate healing. The moxa is normally shaped into a large cigar-like roll, or into small cones. It is then lit and used to send heat and smoke to the skin and acupuncture points to improve the flow of Qi and Blood. This therapy stimulates the acupuncture points and meridians with heat, thus helping to move the Blood and Qi, opening blockages in the body. In addition to the heat created by burning, moxa is also considered a 'Warm' herb, and is thus particularly good for treating 'Cold' conditions and stagnation caused by Cold.[10]

Food Therapy

You are what you eat! This is common sense among Chinese people, just as it is among Westerners. Not only does food have positive or adverse effects on the body in the sense of nutrition, but by definition food also has medicinal impact. A Chinese proverb says, 'Food is medicine and medicines are food'. For the ancient Chinese, there was never a clear-cut distinction between the two.

Rice, ginger, chicken, and lamb are all common foods, but they are also used for their respective medicinal

---

[10]Again, the principles of 'Hot' and 'Cold' will be explored in more detail in chapters to come.

properties. This view was in fact also shared by Hippocrates, who said, 'Let food be thy medicine and medicine be thy food'.

In Chinese herbal medicine, all herbs are classified into 'Hot' and 'Cold' categories, and the same distinction is made with foods. Each type of food is suitable for a certain type of body: 'Cold' food is suitable for a 'Hot' type and 'Hot' food for a 'Cold' type. After a consultation, Chinese doctors will normally tell you what type you fall into, and dietary advice will follow this concept of Hot or Cold. The degree and location of the Hot and the Cold differ, however, with different people, and advice on the level or strength of heating or cooling in the diet follows from a TCM doctor's assessment of each body's relative needs.

Exercise Therapy

Forms of exercise therapy include Qi Gong and Tai Chi, both of which are now popular in the West as well as China. These two exercise therapies are similar, and both involve certain physical movements, control of one's breathing, and meditation. Qi Gong, however, is more static and meditative, while Tai Chi involves more physical movement. Gong Fu or Martial Arts (as depicted in Bruce Lee's movies!) is yet another type which has its followers in the West. This is the most physical, combative, and competitive form of exercise.

Chinese exercises are, in general, different from modern muscular or cardiovascular exercises. They are more connected with the idea of balancing Qi and Blood, as well as using meditation and self-discipline to enhance the well-being of the body. In the Chinese tradition, it is believed that we, as human beings, can learn from other animals, and from their style of movement to better promote health, strength, and energy. Hence, most exercise movements take their inspiration from those of animals, while the *kind* of exercise a patient should attempt follows from the advice of a TCM doctor: who caters their directions to the properties of a patient's body.

Part Three: A Brief History of TCM

For the purposes of this study, it is convenient to divide the history of TCM into three phases.

Antiquity (The Formation of TCM)

TCM coalesced from a set of disparate folk traditions into a semi-coherent body of knowledge and practice over the course of the first phase — from c. 5000 B.C. to approximately 300 B.C.

Some have speculated that our ancestors first created a form of primitive medicine in their struggle against nature: to better survive and to extend that life through the preservation of health. Over the centuries, practitioners accumulated experience in medical knowledge, gradually developing therapeutic methods such as herbal medicine, acupuncture, moxibustion, and medical massage for the prevention and treatment of diseases.

In the period between about 5000 B.C. and 300 B.C., the territory we now call China was in a state of constant internal conflict and instability, with many wars fought between one small state and another. Cultures within China were also divided, from North to South, and state to state, with people holding faith in a variety of gods and legends. As political unification of this territory took place, philosophy, literature, language, and medical thought also became more unified. In around 500 B.C. two great sages emerged: Lao Zi and Kong Zi (Confucius). Their respective philosophies grew to become incredibly influential and went on to dominate all parts of Chinese life, politics, and culture: medicine and health included.

In medicine, the ideas and practices connected with ancient 'Wu Shu' (fortune telling) and other primitive practices came to be replaced by a more naturalistic, body-focused, and less spirit-based medical practice. This development is clearly seen with the generation of the *Yellow Emperor's Canon of Medicine* (*Huang Di Nei Jing*, or *Nei Jing* for short): a medical text produced roughly 2000 years ago.[11]

---

[11] Although scholars are certain the text predates the Han Dynasty, its author and date of composition have been lost to history.

This work can be seen as marking the beginning of the era of TCM proper. It introduces the basic tenants of TCM, covering the theories of Yin–Yang and the Five Elements, 'Zang-Xiang' (organs and their functions), and 'Qi' theory (the production, circulation, and function of internal energy). It also records the 14 main meridian pathways, the locations of the acupuncture points in the body, and acupuncture and moxibustion techniques. It deals at length with the anatomy, physiology, and pathology of the human body, and with the diagnosis, treatment, and prevention of disease. The *Nei Jing* laid a primary foundation for the theories of TCM. Today, it is widely regarded as the 'Bible' of TCM and remains one of its most prominent works of reference.

During the period of the Han Dynasty (about 220 B.C.–220 A.D.), and shortly after the *Nei Jing*, the first work on the 'Materia Medica' (or Chinese Medicines) was compiled: now referred to as *The Herbal Classic of the Divine Ploughman* (*Shen Nong Ben Cao Jing*). This text not only describes the properties and flavours of different herbs but also introduces a classification system that distinguishes their various actions, as either 'Jun' ('emperor'), 'Chen' ('minister'), 'Zuo' ('adjuvant'), or 'Shi' ('messenger') herbs. The distinction between these types, and the logic of their application, is explored later in this text.

The Golden Eras

The 'Golden Eras' refer to the period from around 200 B.C. to 1600 A.D., the early part of which corresponds roughly to the period of the Roman Empire in the West. About 200 years after the time of Lao Zi and Kong Zi, China was united as a single empire, and during the following two millennia, TCM matured and developed across the region. Against this backdrop of greater unification, internal conflicts continued, and there were many dynastic changes over these millennia. Similarly, Traditional Chinese medicine became more refined, even as successive regional variants emerged.

On the shared basis of the theory of the *Nei Jing*, there developed different schools of TCM. These different schools interpreted the *Nei Jing* in various ways, stressing one aspect over another, just as in the West, schisms resulted in different branches of Christianity interpreting the Bible in different ways. These different schools of TCM — and the debates among and between them — greatly enriched and expanded the theories and practice of the tradition, producing many grandmasters who had a lasting influence on the history of world medicine.

1. In the Eastern Han Dynasty (25–220 A.D.), a famous doctor named Zhang Zhong Jing (150–219 A.D.) wrote a text now called the *Treatise on Febrile Diseases and Miscellaneous Diseases*. It was the first to propose diagnosis and treatment based on an overall analysis of signs and symptoms (also called 'pattern differentiation') and laid the foundation for the development of clinical medicine. Altogether, it contains 269 prescriptions for various illnesses.

2. In the Eastern Han Dynasty, the celebrated doctor and surgeon Hua Tao (140–208 A.D.) used a herbal decoction called 'Ma Fei San' to anaesthetise patients, even developing the skill to perform brain surgery! His story was recorded in the famous novel, *The Romance of the Three Kingdoms*, which has been read in China for centuries.

3. The scholar Huang Fu Mi (215–282 A.D.), who lived during the Three Kingdoms period (220–280 A.D.) and Western Jin (265–316 A.D.) Dynasties, compiled the first classic devoted to acupuncture and moxibustion, now called *The A to B Classics of Acupuncture and Moxibustion*. The text addresses channels and collaterals, acupuncture points, acupuncture manipulation, and the indications and contraindications for different acupuncture sites. It remains an influential work and is still frequently consulted by modern acupuncturists.

4. In the Tang Dynasty (618–907 A.D.), the great physician Sun Simiao (581–682 A.D.) devoted his life to two great works, the *Prescriptions for Emergencies Worth a Thousand Pieces of Gold* and *A Supplement to Prescriptions for Emergencies Worth a Thousand Pieces of Gold*. These two works contain over 7000 prescriptions (!) and deal with acupuncture and moxibustion, medicated diets, prevention of disease, and health preservation.

5. Between the 9th and 14th centuries, in the Song and Jin-Yuan Dynasties, there appeared many schools of

herbal medicine, each with their own special features, treatment principles, and herbal formulae. The school of 'Cold' and 'Cool' employed mainly herbs of a Cold or Cool nature in the treatment of febrile diseases. The school of 'Attacking' and 'Purging' used herbs to clear toxins by methods which included diaphoresis, emesis, and purgation, depending on where the toxins were located. The school of 'Nourishing the Earth' involved invigorating the 'Spleen' and 'Stomach' as the main treatment principle. And the school of 'Nourishing the Essence' involved nourishing the 'Essence' and 'Body Waters' to balance excessive 'Fire' in the body.

6. Li Shizhen (1518–1593 A.D.), a great physician of the Ming Dynasty (1368–1644 A.D.), made a huge contribution to the classification of Chinese medicinal herbs. He was a formidable naturalist, and a kind of Chinese Charles Darwin. At first, the personal doctor to the Ming Emperor, he later resigned, returning home to concentrate on the study of herbs. For the rest of his life, he collected, tasted, and experimented on Chinese flora. Among many works, his most important contribution was the vast *Compendium of Materia Medica* (*Ben Cao Gang Mu*), a work which took 27 years to complete and provides details on more than 1800 natural medicines. It was received by scholars of the day as one of the most comprehensive and influential pharmacological works ever written.[12]

---

[12]Li Shizhen was born twenty miles from my hometown in Hubei province. When I was young, there were local herbalists studying

7. Later in the Ming era, TCM scholars discovered a form of immunisation for smallpox. Primitive immunisation methods are recorded which involve giving clothes that had been worn by patients with the disease to those who have never had it, lightly exposing naive patients to a weak form of the illness, providing their immune systems the opportunity to develop immunity. These techniques predated the inoculation work of Edward Jenner by hundreds of years.

Decline and Renaissance

The third period dates from about 300 years ago through to the present. In this period, Western science and medicine were introduced to China, and Chinese medicine faced challenges and competition in all fields.

Western medicine first appeared in China as early as the 16th century, introduced mainly by Christian missionaries. They translated certain Western natural science and medical treatises into Chinese and began performing certain Western medical treatments. One of the most renowned missionaries was Matteo Ricci (1552–1610 A.D.), an Italian Jesuit from the region

---

herbs in their natural environment in a way similar to Li Shizhen. At the age of 13, I was sent by my father to learn herbal medicine from such local medicine men, and thus I was able to participate in a tradition that reached directly back to this great physician and naturalist, 400 years prior.

of Marche.[13] In 1601, Ricci was invited by the Ming Emperor Wan Li to advise the imperial court, as the first Westerner to ever set foot in the Forbidden City.

Gradually, the work of these early missionaries started to influence Chinese culture, science, and indeed medicine. Over time, techniques percolated down from the elite — and soon ordinary people began to experience elements of Western medicine.

In some cases, these practices yielded 'better' results — with patients recovering more quickly when compared with the generally slow results of TCM. Faith in Western medicine began to take hold, and with it, a new social scepticism towards the tenants and methods of TCM. Even within the community of TCM scholars, some physicians began to question its universality. A notable example was the Qing Dynasty TCM doctor Wang Qin Ren (c. 1768–1831 A.D.). Wang took up the Western field of anatomy, dissecting human cadavers and concluding from his research that the organ theory of TCM was wrong. The result was a text titled *The Correction of TCM (Yi Ling Gai Chou)*.

The study of Western medicine developed during the 19th century. Successive Chinese governments started to build Western medicine training centres, and by the

---

[13]350 years after Ricci's birth, I would have the honour to lecture on TCM in Marche, completing a cycle of knowledge exchange that began all those centuries ago!

beginning of the 20th century, there were more schools for Western medicine than for TCM. By the time I formally began my own studies in Guangzhou, there were more than 100 Western medicine colleges and fewer than the 30 TCM colleges in the whole of China.

Many Western-trained Chinese doctors and scientists challenged TCM theories and therapies: TCM was frequently criticised, accusations of its being a pseudo-science followed — and some even pressed for the government to ban TCM altogether.

This current of thought remains strong in parts of the country to this day. There was great urban hostility towards TCM by the time of the first Chinese republican government, and this hostility continued into the early communist period. By 1912, the officially approved government curriculum for medical schools excluded any Chinese medical content. In 1929, a bill was drawn up 'to abolish the old medicine and to clear away obstacles to health'.[14] In 1949, communist health minister Dr. Wang Bing, a surgeon, called TCM a 'feudal medicine'. However, the various attempts to ban TCM failed, and it survived for two simple reasons. First, TCM remained a deep-rooted cultural belief

---

[14] The bill to abolish TCM was proposed by some members of the Health Committee in the Chinese National Health Ministry in February 1929. It caused strong nationwide protests and in March 1929 the bill failed to pass. Hence, the 17th of March is the national TCM Day to remember this event.

among the Chinese people, especially in culturally con-servative, rural areas. Second, it was not practically possible for the Chinese health service to replace TCM with Western medicine. Given the size of the Chinese population, the whole of the Western drug industry would not have been sufficient to supply it.

The renaissance of TCM came with a new policy initi-ated by the Chinese Communist party in the 1950s, which decided to 'combine TCM and Western medicine to serve the people'.[15]After decades of government neglect, by 1956, four new TCM colleges had been established — and this number gradually increased to the current figure of thirty, all of which are funded by the government. At the same time, TCM hospitals were set up in almost all cities and counties in China.[16] I was one of the beneficiaries of this renaissance, and I able to study TCM in a proper university setting and gain clinical experience in busy TCM hospitals.

At time of writing, the picture remains complex. There have been major efforts by the Chinese government to promote TCM, and it remains popular among segments of the population. However, in academic circles, many scholars continue to look down on TCM: maintaining

---

[15]In August 1950, the first Chinese National Health Congress under the communists was held in Beijing, and Chairman Mao gave a superscription for the Congress to form a unique Chinese health system by combining Western and Chinese Medicines.
[16]There are now roughly 1000 such hospitals across the nation.

that it has achieved little and compares unfavourably with Western medicine. Such critics argue, for example, that TCM has not produced any new 'great masters' or 'masterworks' since the crisis of TCM at the cusp of modernity. On this point, I would counter there have been many! And this, despite the political challenges and insufficient funding that have dogged the continued development of TCM.

Regardless, I would argue that such blunt 'culture clash' myths do not serve anybody — and in fact take us further from our common goal of furthering holistic understandings of body and health. When unnuanced comparisons of East and West are drawn up, it is frequently done with only one set of standards and methodologies applied. So, while acknowledging the potency of Western medicine, let us sidestep the trap of defending TCM by comparison, and instead look towards exploring the tradition among its own terms, tools, languages, and logics.

Chapter 2

Metaphysics of TCM

Part One: The '0, 1, 2, 3' Metaphor

What makes TCM unique and so different from Western medicine is its guiding philosophy from which the principles of pathology, diagnosis, treatment, and disease prevention are all directly or indirectly derived.

This philosophy arose within the wider context of ancient Chinese thought, consisting of Daoism, Confucianism, and Buddhism,[1] which have influenced Chinese culture for over two thousand years. While Daoism is fundamental to the natural sciences, Confucianism above all concerns itself with the social realm including such topics as the nature of humanity, justice, social responsibility, and social harmony. Some in China have joked that this mix of philosophies stands

---

[1]Buddhist thought originated in India, but came to China around 200 A.D., where it blended with other currents of Chinese philosophy, and developed into a new 'Chinese' Buddhism, for example in the form of Zen Buddhism.

like shops on a high street: Confucianism, as it serves our daily material needs, is the grocery shop; Daoism, which relates to the scientific and medical quarter, is the pharmacy; and Buddhism, which teaches a little about everything, is the department store.

It therefore follows that the major influence on TCM is Daoist thought. As this is often regarded as an esoteric and enigmatic subject, I have tried to simplify my description using a metaphor consisting of the numbers '0, 1, 2, 3'.

'0' in Philosophy

What is the meaning of the number 0? This seems, at first, an easy question. Many people will say 0 means 'nothing'. How then is it possible for 1 to follow 0 or, in other words, for something to come from nothing? To solve this metaphysical paradox, ancient thinkers reimagined and reframed 0 to represent 'that which is empty or void'. The 0 symbol can be thought of as a circle drawn around an empty space — anything can be put in that space. The invention of 0, which derived from ancient Indian philosophy, expresses exactly the state of emptiness that must come before everything: before 1, at the start of everything, there is 0.

Similarly, ancient Chinese philosophy, especially Daoism, views the beginning of the universe and the nothingness that comes before everything as 'empty' or 'void'.

Dao is '0' in Chinese Philosophy

The 'Dao' is usually translated as 'way', 'path', 'principle', or 'reason'. All these translations only manage to express part of its fuller meaning. To the question of whether there is something rather than nothing in the universe, the Dao is the answer: it is the ultimate truth of the universe, the causation of all things, infinite, timeless, and eternal, and can never be fully described in words. As Lao Zi (c. 6th century B.C.), the father of Daoism, wrote in *The Classic of the Dao and its Virtue (Dao De Jing)*: "The Dao that can be told is not the eternal Dao; the name that can be told is not the eternal name." In essence, Dao is the '0', the infinite empty space that is the eternal driving force behind existence.

The process of transforming emptiness (Figure 2) into something (Figure 3) is understood as being instantaneous and spontaneous. The emptiness, also called 'Wu', transforms itself into a kind of energy called 'Qi': 0 becomes 1. Qi immediately has two forces, negative and positive, called 'Yin' and 'Yang'. These interact with and transform into each other and eventually, through countless transformations, generate all things, including living things and human beings. This process is also called Dao. Dao is therefore the ground of all grounds, the form of all forms, the force of all forces, and the reason of all reasons.

This Daoist doctrine is a kind of ancient materialism. Although both Daoism and Buddhism share the idea of an empty universe, there are some key differences. The Buddhist view is that the world is absolutely empty, and only our minds make it real so that everything you see is in fact a kind of illusion. This doctrine is similar to some versions of Western idealism, as it developed toward existentialism, beginning with Descartes' famous aphorism "I think, therefore I am."

Buddhism believes the world was, is, and will remain empty: that our mind/spirit/soul creates everything, good and bad, and that the soul is reincarnated after death.

In contrast, the Daoist view is that the world was empty to begin with and is now real, but it will be empty again, and real again, then empty again and so on in a process of endless transformation. We could also say that in summation it is half empty and half real. The Dao is not static, it comes and goes without time, and it is this state of change that is absolute. The forces of Yin and Yang can never be perfectly balanced, and this constant state of imbalance will cause constant change.

'1' is Qi

After '0' there is '1'. The ancient Greeks did not consider 1 to be a number at all. Euclid defined a 'number' as an 'aggregate of units', so 1 is not so much a number itself as the essential 'unit' of all numbers. Similarly, in TCM, 'Qi' is the most basic element of the body and of life. In some texts, Qi is known as 'Tai Ji': 'Tai' means 'bigger than big', or the biggest, and 'Ji' means 'ultimate', so together 'Tai Ji' means the ultimate first thing.

'2' is Yin and Yang

Although '1' is the basis and the start, it is only what we rationally infer must exist at the beginning. In Daoism, nothing actually exists as '1': as a single entity. The force or Qi instantly encompasses two opposite parts: Yin and Yang.[2] Everything in the world comes from Qi and everything can be divided into Yin and Yang. These in turn bind to form other things, with the nature of these things depending on how Yin and Yang bind together. In fractal degrees, from the microscopic to the interstellar,[3] Yin and Yang (Figure 4) are constantly intersecting, interacting, and interchanging: leading to a universal state of flux, persistent at all levels.

'3' is a Real Being

The '0-1-2-3' metaphor is summarised by Lao Zi in *Dao De Jing*. He says:

"The Dao begot one, one begot two, two begot three, and three begot the ten thousand things; the ten

---

[2] This neatly mirrors contemporary models of quantum physics, in which each subatomic particle constituting matter is countered by an equal and opposing particle constituting anti-matter. Such parallels, drawing comparison between aspects of ancient Daoist thought and modern particle science, have often been noted and are explored extensively in Fritjof Capra's 1975 text *The Tao of Physics*.

[3] The 'fractal' nature of this phenomena — as it relates to our bodies, and when properly balanced, to our health — is explored in Chapter 7.

thousand things carry Yin and embrace Yang and through their blending of forces achieve harmony."

Yin and Yang, or '2', has a beginning and an end but requires a third dimension to be brought into reality and to create the tangible (Figure 5). For example, an object has length, width, and height; time has past, present, and future; and human society has me, you, and them. In the human body, the interaction of Yin and Yang forms our observable physical body, as 'Jing' and 'Qi': Jing is the 'essence' or the material base of the body and Qi is the live or energetic function of the body. These form a third, more refined, and subtle ability, 'Shen', which does not have an obvious physical form — this can be translated into the mind or 'spirit' of the body and includes its moral values, its knowledge, and its wisdom. The Jing, Qi, and Shen therefore form the basic triadic components of the human body.[4]

The same metaphor appears in the most ancient of Chinese texts on cosmology and philosophy: the *I Ching* (or *Yì Jīng*, often translated as *The Book of Changes*). This text uses a system of symbols to identify the order in chance events and describes what the symbols represent. The symbols are called 'trigrams' (guà) and 'hexagrams.' Each trigram is a figure composed of three stacked horizontal lines (yáo), where each line is either Yang (an unbroken or solid line) or

---

[4]The nature of this triadic unity, as it relates to health through harmonisation, is also addressed in Chapter 7.

Yin (a broken line with a gap in the centre).[5] There are eight possible trigrams. Combining two trigrams forms a hexagram as shown in Figure 1 with six such lines stacked from bottom to top, with 64 possible hexagrammatical combinations.

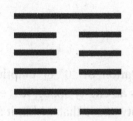

Fig. 1. One of the 64 possible hexagrams in the *I Ching*. Traditionally, hexagram #4 combines the trigram 'Gen' (Yang, Yin, Yin) with 'Kan' (Yin, Yang, Yin).

According to the *I Ching*, these 64 hexagrams represent all possible outcomes of chance events. In the trigram, one can again see this '0-1-2-3' metaphor: without any lines present, there is emptiness, i.e., '0', one line represents 'Qi', i.e., '1', two lines represent Yin and Yang, i.e., '2', and three lines together represent all real and tangible things, i.e., '3' (see Figures 2–5).

The following are some illustrations of Qi or Taiji ('1'), Yin and Yang ('2'), and the trigram with its eight combinations and hexagrams with 64 combinations ('3' or everything).

---

[5]In this context, the Yin and Yang act like the short and long pulses in Morse Code or, in modern terms, like binary constituents of computer 'bytes': constructing meaning, in a dialectical fashion, out of a progressive architecture.

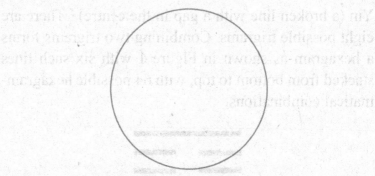

Fig. 2.   A representation of '0' or emptiness. We cannot see anything because it is an empty space. It is exactly because of the existence of this empty space that within it all things can form.

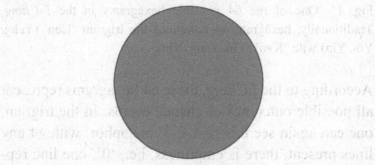

Fig. 3.   A representation of '1'. From nothingness to something, but it is still vague and indivisible.

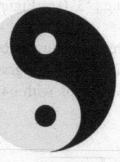

Fig. 4.   A representation of '2'. From a vague form comes the formation of something, with two parts or two dimensions: positive/negative, front/back, inside/outside, light/shadow.

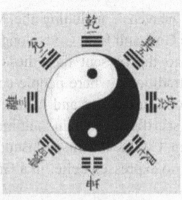

Fig. 5. A representation of '3' or everything. After the appearance of two dimensions, a third dimension arises, here depicted as three lines: broken/unbroken, Yin/Yang. In the combinations made possible by this next dimension, reality begins.

Part Two: Materialism Versus Idealism

Across the ancient world, materialism and idealism arose as the two major metaphysical views of the universe, from Greece and the Near East through to China.

Idealism

As a philosophical position, idealism believes that the fundamental reality of the universe is that of the mind or soul rather than of 'matter'. It also encompasses the belief that the mind controls and can exist independently of the body and that the gods are its creators. Human life is ultimately dependent on the will of the divine.

In ancient Chinese idealism, the view of the gods was polytheistic. These Chinese gods were the 'great divine beings in the heavens', including the Mountain God, Sea God, Tree God, and Rain God, alongside many others. Through to the present day, these gods exist in Chinese folk traditions, where people continue to pray to them for good prosperity and health, believing that good deeds or sacrifices will gain their blessing and protection. Daoism, Confucianism, and Buddhism[6] differ in that they hold no expressed belief in a God or gods.

In opposition to the gods stand demons or evil spirits. In ancient Chinese idealism, demons are the cause of misfortune, including ill health. To resist this, people would pray to the gods in supplication — appealing to divine powers for help exorcising evil spirits — or would treat folk 'witch doctors'[7] and mystics to perform religious healing rituals. TCM, it should be understood, differs radically from such beliefs and practises.

Materialism

Opposing such idealist metaphysics is the materialist view that the reality of the world *is* its material nature, that 'matter' is meaning, and that meaning must in turn

---

[6]As addressed earlier, Buddhism differs slightly in the sense that it advocates for an idealist metaphysical position through the belief that the world is empty, and that only our minds or souls make it real.

[7]While at times dangerously orientalist, this particular phrase can help us by rendering an accurate sense of the synthesis of 'magic', 'religion', and 'medicine' that some early belief systems would invest in such folk healers and their practises.

relate back to 'matter'. In this mode of thought, both body and mind[8] are merely functions of that matter.

Traditional Chinese materialists faced the question that continues to harry modern philosophers: If God(s) did not create matter, what is its origin? As we have seen, with the emergence of Lao Zi around 2500 years ago, with the seminal work *Dao De Jing*, a materialist solution was found, which did not, by its definition, require theistic or idealistic attributes.[9]

The development of Daoist materialism profoundly affected Chinese culture reshaping traditional understandings of the natural world and leaving its mark on TCM philosophy.

At times, this materialist view has been tarnished by deliberate hands, as when fringe medical practitioners mix TCM with certain spiritual practises. At times, it is accidentally undermined, as when poor translation of ancient texts misrepresents elements of TCM as spiritual in nature. Yet, at its core, since the rise of Daoism, TCM has belonged to a fundamentally materialist worldview.

---

[8] And, therefore, the 'health' of either or both.

[9] This is not to say that certain Daoist materialist traditions did not, at times, include these elements, and certainly, many practitioners of materialistic thought would also subscribe to regional idealistic beliefs or rituals, rather it is enough to note that Daoist materialism does not require God or gods to resolve the question of existence.

A religious form of Daoism did also develop, around 600 years after Lao Zi, during the Eastern Han Dynasty. Folk traditions began to use Daoist philosophy to deify Lao Zi: building Daoist temples complete with images and statues of his likeness and generating folk myths and rituals out of his legend. Out of such neotheologicality followed a belief that, just as the Dao itself is eternal, people too might obtain immortality. Believers, among them — Daoist monks — meditated on the Dao, hoping to become enlightened. Some of these forms of meditation, especially Transcendental Meditation, are known by many in the West today. For our purposes, it is important to remember that Daoism at its core is a materialistic philosophy, and we should make a clear distinction between Daoism and subsequent Daoist religion.[10]

TCM, too, belongs to the philosophical tradition and is not part of the Daoist religion.

TCM therefore addresses body and mind without acknowledging the soul as a separate entity. The mind extends from the function of our organs, especially the

---

[10]It is regrettable that the theological legacies of Daoism have obstructed its philosophical origins in this way, such that, to the Western imagination, Daoist philosophy and Daoist religion are muddied and intermixed. Therefore, when explaining the origin and reasoning of TCM to the Western reader, it is important to attempt a deprogramming: to separate out the Daoist materialism once again, we have studied here — which sincerely influenced Traditional Chinese Medicine — from the Daoist religion, that many Westerners may have seen glimpses of in meditation classes or popular culture.

function of the heart.[11] In this sense, traditional Chinese philosophy is consistent with that of modern Western medicine, which considers the mind as a function of the body without supernatural dynamics. Chinese medicine only differs in associating the mind with the heart, whereas Western medicine traditionally attributes the mind to the function of the brain.[12]

TCM, therefore, adopts the same metaphysical framework as Western medicine, and perhaps this is partly why TCM has survived for so long alongside it.

Part Three: Holism

Another central idea in TCM is that of 'holism', that we should understand the whole holistically rather than as a sum of disparate parts. As ancient TCM thinkers turned away from a supernatural understanding of the

---

[11] Incidentally, this is why, in Chinese, one will often find phrases such as 'thinking with your heart', 'good-hearted man', or 'bad-hearted man'.

[12] Mainstream Western tradition, from the *Corpus Hippocraticum* (c. 4th century BC) through to Descartes (c. 17th century), the Enlightenment (c. 18th century), and the conventional wisdom of our present time, has consistently located the function of 'mind' to the brain. However, in recent decades — and in such a way that neatly demonstrates our argument in Chapter 1 that asked for room to be kept aside for Western science to develop into ground already broken by TCM — much work has been done that complicates this picture. Indeed, many recent studies have explored the importance of other organs in the creation of what TCM and Western doctors both refer to as 'mind'.

human body, they instead sought understanding in the 'natural', making efforts to relate the human body and its functions to the wider world. They observed structure and patterns in nature and reasoned that because the human body is also natural in origin, it might also follow these same structures and patterns. They observed that the constituents of nature relate to one other in ways that form a *whole and* reasoned that the human body must also form a whole, as a microcosm of the wider world.

The classic TCM text, *The Yellow Emperor's Classic of Internal Medicine (Huang Di Nei Jing)*, argues that the Earth is crested with two shining spheres, just as we humans have two eyes; the Earth has mountains, as the body has bones; the Earth has rivers, as it has blood; and the Earth is spotted with trees and grass, as the surface of our skin is quilted in hair.

As this 'holistic' method is key to understanding the logic of TCM, this section will explore the core ways in which the human body, *as* whole, reflects the holistic elements of the natural world.

The Five Elements Theory
Today, we understand that the building blocks of the universe are the chemical elements of the periodic table, but in the ancient world, this knowledge had not

yet been fully embraced. Instead, people categorised things based on what they could see. In Europe and India, they concluded that there were four basic elements; in China, scholars concluded there were five: Fire, Water, Wood, Metal, and Earth.

As illustrated in Table 1, the 'Five Elements Theory' explores how these elements connect with and correspond to various concepts in nature, including the organs of the human body. The theory is commonly used to analyse disease pathology and to guide

Table 1.   Correspondence of the Five Elements.

	Wood	Fire	Earth	Metal	Water
Directions	East	South	Centre	West	North
Climates	Wind	Heat	Dampness	Dryness	Cold
Seasons	Spring	Summer	Middle summer	Autumn	Winter
Colour	Green	Red	Yellow	White	Black
Tastes	Sour	Bitter	Sweet	Acrid	Salty
Stages of development	Birth	Growth	(Mature) Transform	Harvest	Storage
Musical notes	Me	So	Do	Re	La
Zhang organs (Yin)	Liver	Heart	Spleen	Lung	Kidney
Fu organs (Yang)	Gallbladder	Small intestine	Stomach	Large intestine	Bladder
Sense organs	Eyes	Tongue	Mouth	Nose	Ears
Tissues	Sinews	Vessels	Muscles	Skin	Bones
Emotions	Anger	Joy	Pensiveness	Sadness	Fear
Sounds	Shouting	Laughing	Singing	Crying	Groaning

treatments in TCM and still has wide applications in many other areas of life and society in China.

Fire

Fire corresponds to the summer season. It is associated with heat and the provision of energy. In TCM, the organ characterised by Fire is the Heart, which controls the circulation of blood and provides energy and warmth to the body.

Water

Water irrigates, moisturises, cleanses, and purifies. In TCM, the organ characterised by Water is the Kidney, which controls the irrigation of the body, providing nourishment to the body while ceaselessly cleansing bodily systems. All living things are dependent on water. Similarly, in TCM, the Kidney is the 'root' of the human body.

Wood

Wood corresponds to the season of spring and is associated with birth and growth. Trees and grasses grow quickly in spring and can be bent or straightened depending on their resilience. The internal organ that is characterised by Wood is the Liver, which provides for the nutrition of the body through blood.

Metal

Metals are hard and solid and, in TCM, are connected to ripening and hardening grains or nuts, therefore corresponding to autumn and the associated harvest. In TCM, the organ characterised by the Metal is the Lung, the movements of which allow a necessary downward motion of circulating Qi and Water, like the falling grains and fruits of autumn.

Earth

Earth, in one school of TCM thought, does not correspond to any season because it is the centre of the universe[13] or the neutral term of reference around which the seasons and elements spin. In another school of thought, the Earth corresponds to the 'Late Summer Season', which is the period after the summer solstice and before the early part of autumn. Earth, often called Mother Earth, permits sowing, growing, reaping, and the provision of nourishment by nature. The corresponding organ in the body is the Spleen, as it is believed to control the digestion and absorption of food and water.

Part Four: Interrelationships of the Five Elements

The Five Elements do not exist as separate parts but in dynamic interunion; in every material state, they interact through movement and change. This change is far

---

[13]Ancient people in China, and in the West, thought that the Earth was the centre of the universe and that the sun, moon, and stars circled the Earth.

from chaotic but instead obeys principles that, with a holistic approach, can be used to understand the organs and bodies the elements constitute.

The principles that underlie every holistic form include the following:

The Generating Sequence

When one element promotes another, this is called 'mutual generation' or the 'generating sequence' (Figure 6). For example, Wood promotes Fire, Fire promotes Earth, Earth promotes Metal, Metal promotes Water, and Water promotes Wood. In nature, we often observe this kind of mutual generation: wood can be burnt to produce fire; after the fire burns out, then ash becomes earth; within earth, metals are formed and found; metals can be borne in liquid solutions to nourish trees and wood. In TCM, this sequence is sometimes expressed in terms of a 'mother' and 'child' relationship: for example, 'Wood is the Child of Water and the Mother of Fire' or 'Water is the Mother of Wood and the Child of Metal', etc.

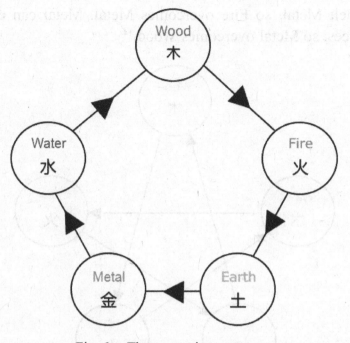

Fig. 6.　The generating sequence.

The Controlling Sequence

In opposition to the 'generating sequence' is the 'controlling sequence' (Figure 7). This is when the Five Elements control and restrain each other: Wood overcomes Earth, Earth overcomes Water, Water overcomes Fire, Fire overcomes Metal, and Metal overcomes Wood. Again, in nature, we might notice trees grow out of the Earth, so Wood overcomes Earth. Earth stops water or flooding, so Earth overcomes Water. Water extinguishes Fire, so Water overcomes Fire. Fire can melt Metal, so Fire overcomes Metal. Metal can cut trees, so Metal overcomes Wood.[14]

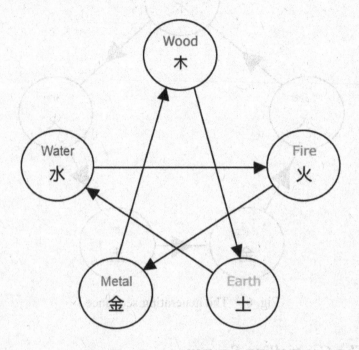

Fig. 7.   The controlling sequence.

[14]There also exists a balancing interrelationship of *negative feedback* between the generating and controlling sequences. For instance, Wood controls Earth, but Earth generates Metal which in turn controls Wood. Additionally, Wood controls Earth, but Wood also generates Fire which in turn generates Earth. This illustrates a self-regulating balance or homeostasis maintained in nature, including in the human body. Interestingly, homeostasis is a key holistic aspect of Western medicine — and here, again, we can observe the fundamental commonalities between the two traditions, as both observe the importance of negative feedback loops in the pursuit of balance within the body. This is explored in greater detail in Chapter 7.

The Overacting Sequence

Sometimes, balance between the elements is not maintained. One element can overcontrol another (Figure 8), resulting in a relative excess of one element over another. For example, in normal circumstances, Fire controls Metal, but if Fire is too strong and 'overcontrols' Metal, Metal becomes relatively weak and cannot properly generate Water. This in turn causes a deficiency in Water which can further weaken its control on the already overacting Fire.

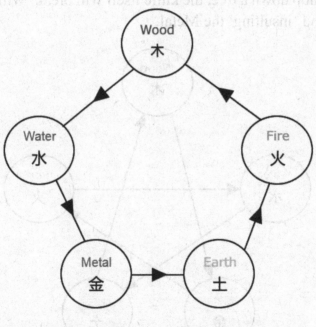

Fig. 8.   The overacting sequence.

The Insulting Sequence

The 'insulting sequence' (Figure 9) is the 'controlling sequence' but in reverse order. Again, this takes place when a disruption to the self-regulating balance of the elements occurs. For instance, Water usually controls Fire, but in abnormal conditions if the Water has dried up, this can permit a reversal of the usual sequence and Fire then controls, or 'insults', Water.

In another analogy, while Metal usually controls Wood, if a small piece of metal, such as a kitchen knife, tries to chop down a tree, the knife itself will break! With the Wood 'insulting' the Metal.

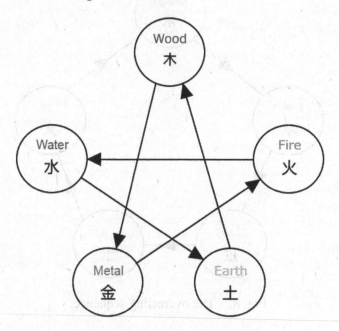

Fig. 9. The insulting sequence.

In order to demonstrate the overall complexity of Five Elements theory and the interrelationships of the elements, it is useful to show the sequences overlaid as a composition (Figure 10).

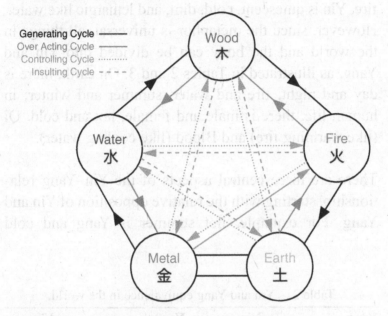

Fig. 10. Composite image of the Five Elements sequences.

Part Five: Yin and Yang in the Human Body

In Daoism, as explored earlier, Yin and Yang together represent a fundamental dualism of the universe and the 'whole' as well as the bipolar, oscillating cycles of nature. Accordingly, because the human body is part of the universe and part of nature, its physiology and pathology can similarly be reduced to Yin and Yang.

In Chinese, Yang literally means the sun or something facing sunlight, while Yin literally means the moon or shade. The ancient Chinese mostly used the examples of water and fire: Yang is hot, bright, and hyperactive like fire, Yin is quiescent, cold, dim, and lethargic like water. However, since the metaphor is universal, all things in the world and the body can be divided into Yin and Yang, as illustrated in Tables 2 and 3. On earth, there is day and night, fire and water, summer and winter; in human life, there is male and female, hot and cold, Qi (like warming fire) and Blood (like cooling water).

There are three central aspects of the Yin–Yang relationship, starting with the relative opposition of Yin and Yang. For example, hot summer is Yang and cold

Table 2.   Yin and Yang equivalence in the world.

Yang	Yin	Yang	Yin
Summer	Winter	Outside	Inside
Heat	Cold	Exterior	Interior
Male	Female	Young	Old
Light	Dark	White	Black
Acute	Chronic	Moving	Static
Up	Down	Happy	Depressed
Sky	Earth	Spicy food	Sweet food
East	West	Red meat	White meat
South	North	High voice	Low voice
Left	Right	Spastic	Flaccid
Fast	Slow		

Table 3. Yin and Yang equivalence in TCM.

Yang	Yin	Yang	Yin
Small intestine	Heart	Qi	Blood
Gallbladder	Liver	Skin and hair	Muscles and bone
Large intestines	Lung	Move	Rest
Stomach	Spleen	Feeling hot	Feeling cold
Urinary bladder	Kidney	Red	Pale
Triple heater	Pericardium	Hyperactivity	Hypoactivity
Head	Body	Short term	Long term
Upper limbs	Lower limbs		

winter is Yin, but even in the hot summer and cold winter, day belongs to Yang and night belongs to Yin.

Second, Yin and Yang are interdependent: one cannot exist without the other, as day cannot exist without night. The mutual consumption of Yin and Yang means that there is a constant state of dynamic balance, which is maintained by continuous adjustments of the relative levels of Yin and Yang.

Third, Yin and Yang are not static, as there is constant intertransformation. Day changes into night and vice versa. Heat from the sun evaporates water to form rain which nurtures living things, while in the human body, the Kidney Yang, also known as the 'inner sun', moves fluids and nutrients to every part of the body to sustain life.

In the familiar symbol of Yin and Yang (Figure 4), the black portion represents Yin and the white portion

Yang. Both are within a single entity, the wider 'whole'. The division between Yin and Yang is not straight but curved, symbolic of the way nature is never straightforward, black, or white, but rather exists in relative shades of grey. Of significance are the smaller circles representing Yin in Yang and Yang in Yin because of the mutual waxing and waning, interdependence and intertransformation. A wholly pure Yin or Yang condition does not exist.

The Five Solid Organs

Like a natural ecosystem, our body houses a complex and complete network of organs and interconnections.

At the core of this network are five organs — five because they imitate and correspond with the Five Elements. These consist of the Heart, Lung, Spleen, Liver, and Kidney, their core role identified because of their location in the centre and innermost parts of the body, hence they are called 'Zang' in Chinese, the literal translation of which is 'hidden' and 'storing'. In structure, they are solid, as opposed to hollow, and so are often also called the 'solid organs'.

It is important to note that though these five organs are given identical names in Western medicine, their meaning is different. This kind of confusion has arisen numerous times in my clinical practise — I have told patients in the past that they had a problem with their

'Kidney' according to their TCM diagnosis, only for them to consult a Western doctor about their kidneys who, unsurprisingly, found nothing wrong with them from their perspective. To be clear, there is some overlap between the meaning of 'Kidney' or any organ in the two medical systems, but in TCM these terms tend to have a broader meaning, referencing whole systems, while Western medicine employs narrower meanings, referencing only single organs.[15] Even beyond this, there are no doubt differences between the meanings of the organs in the two systems. For example, the TCM belief that the five solid organs control and dominate all other parts of the body would be unfamiliar to a Western medicine doctor.

The TCM beliefs about the nature and function of the five solid organs are summarised in the following, and their structural and functional relationships are laid out in tables.

---

[15] From here another common question arises: Why continue to use the ancient concepts rather than switching to the new, more precise concepts? My answer is that although the ancient concepts are a little vague and imprecise, the broader views of the organs and their links with other organs and tissues will enable us to see more clearly the whole picture of the body, allowing doctors to make more holistic treatment plans. In TCM, we believe that the results of such treatment plans are more effective and sustainable than those which target very specific organs only, and clinical practise has taught me that patients care more about results than terminology.

Heart

The heart controls mental activities (i.e., the spirit or 'Shen') and governs the Blood, blood vessels, and meridians.

Houses	Shen or mind
Controls	Sweat
Vital substances	Governs Blood
Tissues	Controls blood vessels and manifests in the complexion
Sense organs	Opens into the tongue and controls taste
Emotions	Relates to joy
Climates	(Adversely) Influenced by Heat

Liver

The liver governs the normal flow of Qi and Blood and unblocks any blockages in the flow. It smooths the distribution of Qi and Blood, especially by storing Blood to regulate its distribution. This helps the heart control the spirit.

Houses	Ethereal soul
Controls	Smooth flow of Qi
Vital substances	Stores Blood
Tissues	Controls sinews and manifests in the nails
Sense organs	Opens into the eyes and controls sight
Emotions	Relates to anger
Climates	(Adversely) Influenced by Wind

Lung

The Lung controls Qi, including the formation of Qi by combining the 'Qi of Heaven' (i.e., air) and our own Qi into our life force, and the dissemination of Qi up and down throughout the body.

Houses	Corporeal soul
Controls	Channels and blood vessels
Controls	Regulation of water passages
Vital substances	Governs Qi respiration and influences body fluids
Tissues	Controls skin and manifests in the body hair
Sense organs	Opens into the nose and controls smell
Emotions	Relates to grief and sadness
Climates	(Adversely) Influenced by Dryness

Spleen

The Spleen dominates the transformation and transportation of food essences, including the digestion and absorption of food and the dissemination of nutrients. It also transforms and transports water and fluids. These make up the basic sources of nourishment for the body.

Houses	Thought
Controls	Raising of Qi
Vital substances	Governs food Qi, holds Blood, and influences body fluids
Tissues	Controls muscles and four limbs and manifests in the lips
Sense organs	Opens into the mouth and controls taste
Emotions	Relates to worry
Climates	(Adversely) Influenced by Dampness

Kidney

The Kidney stores the 'Jing' or 'essence' of the body, the heritable component that is passed from parent to child. At the beginning of new life, this 'original essence' is transformed into Yin and Yang. The resultant Kidney Yin and Yang provide the force required to grow, nurture, warm, and cool. The warming function is important for defending against infections. The cooling function is important for clearing out toxins and metabolic by-products.

Houses	Intelligence and confidence
Controls	Water and urine
Vital substances	Stores essence and influences body fluids
Tissues	Controls bones and manifests in the hair

(*Continued*)

Sense organs	Opens into the ears and controls hearing
Emotions	Relates to fear and confidence
Climates	(Adversely) Influenced by Cold

To illustrate their functions, the organs are sometimes compared to positions in a government: the Heart is the emperor controlling the spirit or 'Shen', the Lung is the premier of the body controlling Qi, the Spleen is the treasurer controlling nutrition, the Liver is the minister of justice keeping the body in a state of harmony, and the Kidney is the minister of defence protecting the body from external invasion by germs and the build-up of internal toxins.

The Five Hollow Organs and Other Subsidiaries

The Small Intestine, Large Intestine, Stomach, Gallbladder, and Urinary Bladder make up the five 'hollow' organs. Compared to the solid organs, they are all located more superficially and do not provide storage, i.e., of the nourishment or 'Jing' (essence). They also sometimes go by their Chinese name, 'Fu', which means 'house' in reference to their hollow structure.

They are paired with the solid organs: the Small Intestine with the Heart, the Large Intestine with the Lung, the Stomach with the Spleen, the Gallbladder with the Liver, and the Urinary Bladder with the Kidney.[16]

Other parts of the body are further subsidiary elements to the solid and hollow organs:

Heart–Small Intestine:	Tongue, blood vessels
Lung–Large Intestine:	Nose, skin, hair of the body
Spleen–Stomach:	Mouth, lips, muscle
Liver–Gallbladder:	Eyes, tendons, ligaments, nails
Kidney–Urinary Bladder:	Ears, bone, marrow, brain, hair of the head

Other subdivisions based on the five solid organs also exist: in Reflexology, the feet are divided into five areas that through massage can help heal the associated organs. For the detailed treatment of eye diseases, the eye itself can also be divided into areas linked with the five organs: the pupil of the eye is linked with the Kidney, the iris with the Lung, the clear surface of the eye, the cornea, with the Liver, the corners of the eye with Heart, and the eyelids with Spleen.

---

[16]While some of these pairings seem clear, others may seem strange to Western eyes. It's important to understand that the pairings arose from historical clinical observations of symptoms and patterns, and in my own clinical practise, I continue to see some of these patterns playing out, e.g., patients with lung problems also complaining of bowel problems.

The Subtle Network of Meridians and Channels

In TCM, there exist connections between organs that are both visible, such as blood vessels, and invisible. The latter are known as Qi channels or 'meridians.' Acupuncture treatment is based on this meridian theory: in our body, there are 14 large meridians, including 12 regular meridians and two special meridians, and many subsidiaries and interconnections. On each meridian, there are key points that are used for acupuncture — we call these 'acupuncture points' or 'acupoints' and there are 365 such acupoints around the body.

A question will be raised here: What about the nervous system? Modern medicine has made clear that the nervous system itself is an important network of connections between organs. Is a meridian, therefore, a nerve? A great deal of thought and research has been and continues to be put into the question of what the meridian system is or represents. Indeed, in TCM, many of the functions of meridians are similar to that of the nervous system, and so far, the conclusion is that the meridian system and the nervous system overlap but are not identical.

In the eyes of the scientific community, there remains doubt over the existence of the meridian system. Although this discussion is beyond the scope of this book, I will add that many doctors even in TCM want to replace the meridian theory with a nervous system theory. My personal opinion is that it is too early to draw a conclusion. I believe the meridian system describes very subtle connections that, like other aspects of the body and also the wider world, are unclear, changeable, and difficult to observe. The nervous system theory itself also has limitations — modern science still struggles to explain the mind and how the mind and body interact. It is for these reasons that I along with the majority of TCM doctors continue to use the meridian theory in clinical practise.

Why are the Yang meridians on the back and outer aspects of the limbs and why are the Yin meridians on the front and inner aspects of the limbs? Imagine an animal walking on all fours; the back and outer aspects of the limbs are exposed to sunlight which corresponds to Yang, while the front and inner aspects of the limbs are in shade which corresponds to Yin.

The 12 regular meridians are connected to 12 organs. Their connections are depicted in the Figures. 11–22:

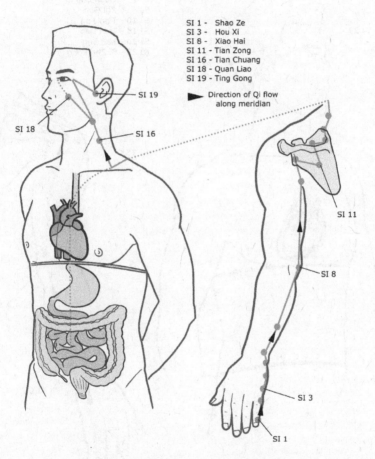

SI 1 - Shao Ze
SI 3 - Hou Xi
SI 8 - Xiao Hai
SI 11 - Tian Zong
SI 16 - Tian Chuang
SI 18 - Quan Liao
SI 19 - Ting Gong

► Direction of Qi flow along meridian

Fig. 11.   Small Intestine Hand Tai Yang Meridian.

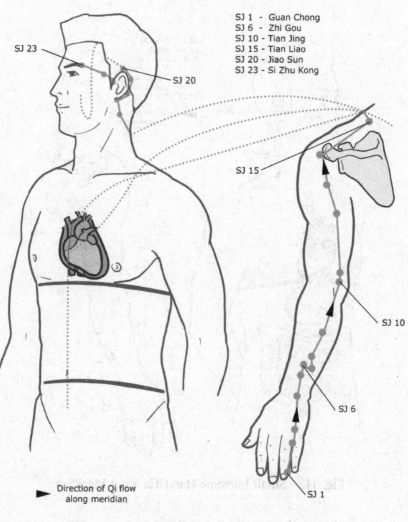

SJ 1 - Guan Chong
SJ 6 - Zhi Gou
SJ 10 - Tian Jing
SJ 15 - Tian Liao
SJ 20 - Jiao Sun
SJ 23 - Si Zhu Kong

SJ 23

SJ 20

SJ 15

SJ 10

SJ 6

SJ 1

► Direction of Qi flow
along meridian

Fig. 12.   San Jiao Hand Shao Yang Meridian.

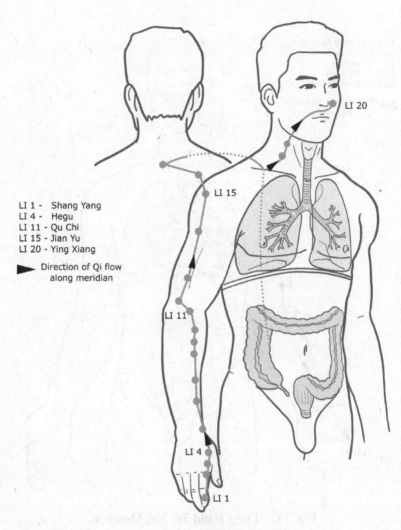

LI 20

LI 15

LI 1 - Shang Yang
LI 4 - Hegu
LI 11 - Qu Chi
LI 15 - Jian Yu
LI 20 - Ying Xiang

► Direction of Qi flow
along meridian

LI 11

LI 4

LI 1

Fig. 13.   Large Intestine Hand Yang Ming Meridian.

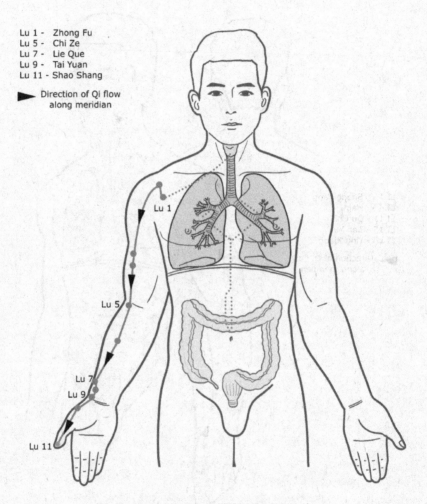

Lu 1 -   Zhong Fu
Lu 5 -   Chi Ze
Lu 7 -   Lie Que
Lu 9 -   Tai Yuan
Lu 11 - Shao Shang

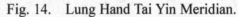 Direction of Qi flow
          along meridian

Fig. 14.   Lung Hand Tai Yin Meridian.

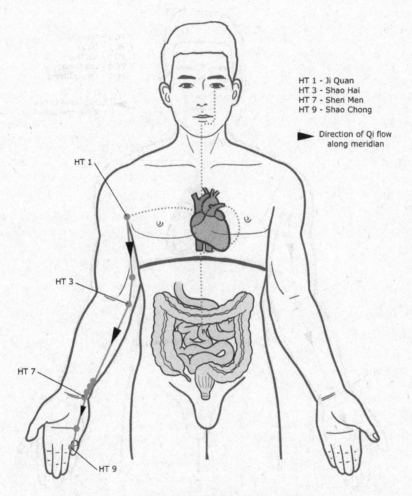

Fig. 15.   Heart Hand Shao Yin Meridian.

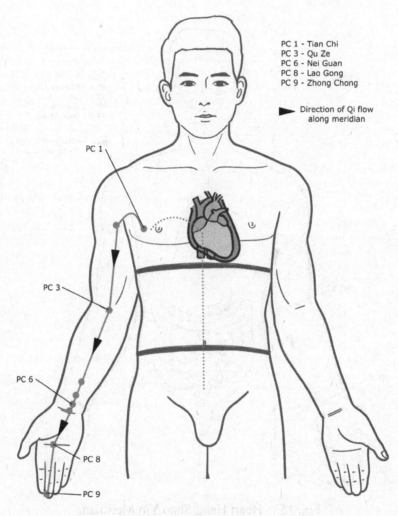

PC 1 - Tian Chi
PC 3 - Qu Ze
PC 6 - Nei Guan
PC 8 - Lao Gong
PC 9 - Zhong Chong

► Direction of Qi flow
along meridian

PC 1

PC 3

PC 6

PC 8

PC 9

Fig. 16.   Pericardium Hand Jue Yin Meridian.

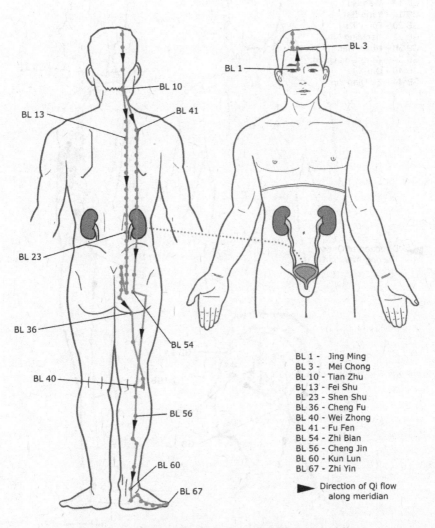

BL 1 - Jing Ming
BL 3 - Mei Chong
BL 10 - Tian Zhu
BL 13 - Fei Shu
BL 23 - Shen Shu
BL 36 - Cheng Fu
BL 40 - Wei Zhong
BL 41 - Fu Fen
BL 54 - Zhi Bian
BL 56 - Cheng Jin
BL 60 - Kun Lun
BL 67 - Zhi Yin

▶ Direction of Qi flow
along meridian

Fig. 17.   Urinary Bladder Foot Tai Yang Meridian.

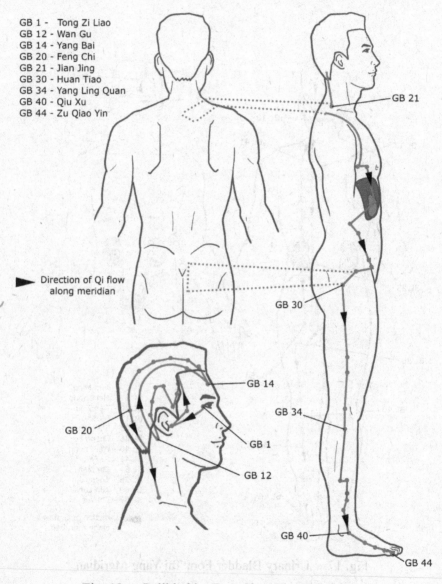

GB 1 -   Tong Zi Liao
GB 12 - Wan Gu
GB 14 - Yang Bai
GB 20 - Feng Chi
GB 21 - Jian Jing
GB 30 - Huan Tiao
GB 34 - Yang Ling Quan
GB 40 - Qiu Xu
GB 44 - Zu Qiao Yin

▶ Direction of Qi flow
along meridian

GB 21

GB 30

GB 14

GB 34

GB 20

GB 1

GB 12

GB 40

GB 44

Fig. 18.   Gallbladder Foot Shao Yang Meridian.

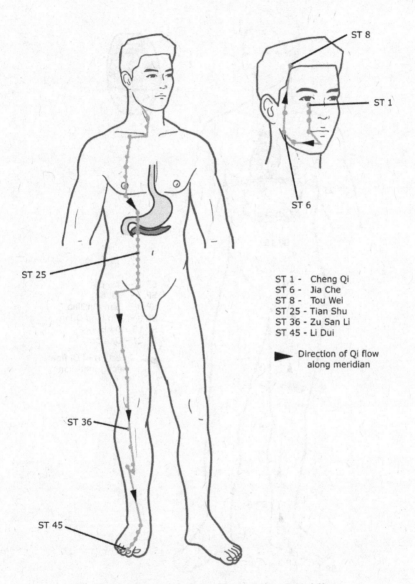

Fig. 19. Stomach Foot Yang Ming Meridian.

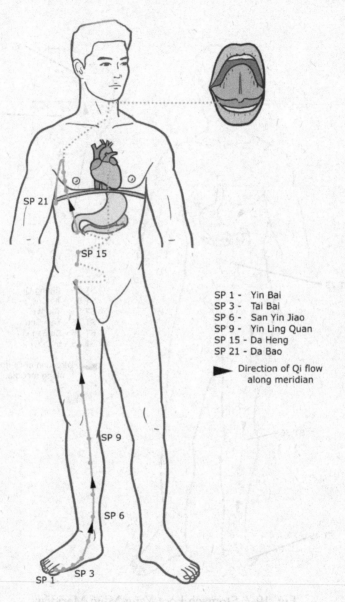

SP 21

SP 15

SP 1 - Yin Bai
SP 3 - Tai Bai
SP 6 - San Yin Jiao
SP 9 - Yin Ling Quan
SP 15 - Da Heng
SP 21 - Da Bao

► Direction of Qi flow
   along meridian

SP 9

SP 6

SP 1 SP 3

Fig. 20.   Spleen Foot Tai Yin Meridian.

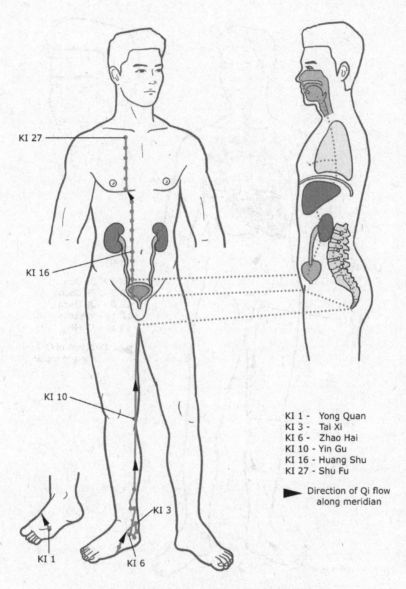

KI 27

KI 16

KI 10

KI 3

KI 1

KI 6

KI 1 - Yong Quan
KI 3 - Tai Xi
KI 6 - Zhao Hai
KI 10 - Yin Gu
KI 16 - Huang Shu
KI 27 - Shu Fu

► Direction of Qi flow
along meridian

Fig. 21. Kidney Foot Shao Yin Meridian.

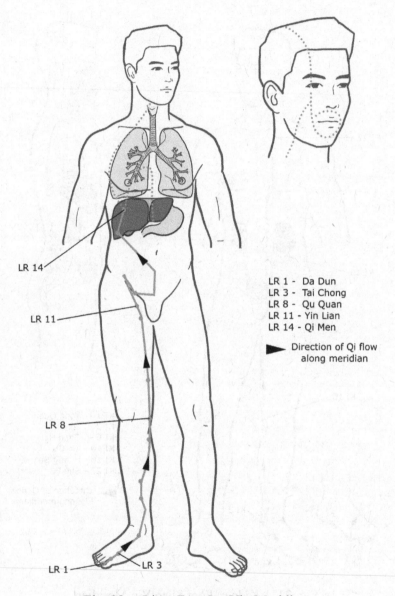

Fig. 22.   Liver Foot Jue Yin Meridian.

TCM doctors often find it difficult to explain what the 'San Jiao' organ is. All other organs in TCM have a corresponding tangible, physical form, but the San Jiao organ does not. Texts describe that it is situated in the thorax and abdomen and is the largest Fu, or hollow, organ in the body; its main function is to move primordial (Yuan) Qi or original Qi and to circulate body fluid. The San Jiao is also unusual in that it is not paired with a Zang organ.

A detailed discussion of this concept goes beyond the scope of this book, but in my personal understanding, San Jiao represents a function, rather than a physical organ, that only emerges when all other organs function actively. 'San' is the number three in Chinese and 'Jiao' means 'burning' — some books therefore translate San Jiao as the 'three burners.' The key here is its active functioning or 'burning' that can only be found in a living body, not a dead one.

The two special meridians are called the 'Du' meridian and the 'Ren' meridian. While the other 12 regular meridians are symmetrically distributed on the right and left sides of the body, the Du and the Ren meridians are on the front and back. The Du meridian begins at the middle of the head, at the upper lip, and then goes to the top of the head and down the back, along the central spinal column to the anus. It governs all the Yang meridians of the body and is often called the sea of all Yang meridians. The Ren meridian begins at the lower lip and goes down to the genitals. It meets all the Yin meridians of the body and governs Blood and body fluid. It is called the sea of all Yin meridians. It is especially important for the genitals or reproductive organs and for women, controlling menstruation, pregnancy, and birth.

Apart from these 14 meridians, 12 regular meridians, and two special meridians, there are many smaller tributaries or 'collaterals' which form tiny networks, like capillaries, all over the body. With these tributaries, the meridian system connects the whole body, from inside to outside, even down to the tiniest cell.

These five Zang organs, their pairing Fu organs, and subsidiary tissues, together with the whole network of meridians, form the complete and unified network that we call the human body. All parts are connected directly or indirectly, forming a holistic unity. They work together as a whole and influence each other for good or, in disease states, for bad.

Chapter 3

Causes of Disease

Unlike other forms of ancient medicine, TCM does not ascribe the causes of illness to supernatural forces such as ghosts, demons, or evil spirits. The causes of illness are material and many and can be divided into external and internal sets.

Part One: External Causes of Disease

Traditionally, the most powerful of external causes are those which consist of natural, environmental changes. At its most primal, such change can be rendered in abnormal weather conditions: dramatic shifts in climate or extreme cold, wind, humidity, or drought. These are summarised as the 'Six Evils',[1] including Wind, Cold, Heat (or Fire), Summer-Heat, Dampness, and Dryness. While these are the most potent of external causes,

---

[1]Although the word 'evils' is most often used in translation, the phrase refers to something harmful rather than implying an unnatural thing or supernatural force.

there are countless others: from insect bites to animal attacks, from burns to injuries to accidents.

The Six Evils

In every environment, the flow of Qi shifts with the seasons: in the plains, it may be hot in summer, while it is dry in the desert and damp in a swamp. According to TCM, there are six basic climatic states that exist in the natural world: Wind, Cold, Summer-Heat, Dampness, Dryness, and Fire. We call these the 'Six Qi'.

Yin and Yang take control alternatively and each dominates the climate in turn. Despite there being many other weather phenomena, all can be classified into one of the Six Qi.

The number six was chosen by the ancient Chinese because they considered the human world as a middle point between Heaven and Earth. Therefore, the Cosmos was divided in six directions, each leading out from this middle kingdom: to the East; West; North; South; above in the sky; and below in the earth. Given the geography of China, it followed that the predominant weather to the 'East' is Wind, to the 'North' is Cold, to the West is Dryness, to the South is Fire, and in the middle is Dampness from the earth and Summer-Heat from the sky.

When changes in weather and Qi occur smoothly, the body can cope and correspondingly adjusts its functions to suit. When the changes are violent, or contrary to season or place, a violent reaction can follow. The climate then becomes pathogenic, and the Six Qi become the Six Evils.

Wind

Wind is considered the first 'Evil' of the Six, because in large parts of China, the wind is strong across all four seasons. It follows that in China, many of the 'external' diseases are associated with Wind: such as Wind-Cold, Wind-Heat, and Wind-Damp syndromes.

If we study wind in nature, we will find that it is characterised by certain features. The symptoms of patients with the Wind 'Evil' bear some hallmarks of these features.

Floating and upwards moving: Wind is a pathogenic factor of a Yang nature, characterised by lightness. That is why Wind attacks the upper part of the body (the head and face) and skin first, and manifests as headaches, sore throats, and runny noses.

Moving: Wind is mobile and the diseases caused by it also migrate, moving around the body: such as the migratory limb pain in so-called 'Wind-Bi' syndrome, a TCM name for a kind of arthritis. This is also articulated in limb tremors (such as shaking, convulsions, or spasm), dizziness, and vertigo. Alongside external Wind 'evil', TCM acknowledges in-kind *internal* Wind evils: such as 'Liver-Wind', a condition caused by Liver dysfunction, which I will discuss later.[2]

Rapid change: Wind tends to change quickly, so the diseases caused by Wind are often characterised by sudden onset, quick change, and rapid transferral into other problems.[3] For example, an initial cold can very easily become pneumonia.

Complications: Wind tends to be complicated by or combined with other pathogenic factors. Since it is easier for Wind to attack the body, other external factors often attach themselves to or follow Wind when invading the body, frequently leading to 'Wind-Cold' syndrome, 'Wind-Heat' syndrome, 'Wind-Dampness' syndrome, and 'Wind-Dryness' syndrome. It follows in this sense too that Wind 'leads' among the Six Evils: where, to some extent, all diseases are initiated by Wind.

Cold

Cold is another common evil, attacking the body frequently, especially in winter, and it should be noted that Central and Northern China experience long winters. The famous TCM text entitled *Treatise on Febrile Diseases and Miscellaneous Diseases* (*Shang Han Lun*) by Dr. Zhang Zhong Jing (150 A.D.–219 A.D.)

---

[2] This condition of Liver-Wind will be discussed in the *Liver Syndromes* of Chapter 5.

[3] As well as a quick recovery — if dealt with properly!

specifically addresses Cold's effects on the body. Prescriptions from this book are still used daily in our clinical practice. In fact, between the years 2020 and 2022, Chinese hospitals have been using some of its prescriptions — or variations thereof — to treat COVID-19 infections countrywide.

Cold tends to impair Yang: By its nature, Cold pertains to Yin and tends to impair Yang. When Cold takes hold on the surface of the body, it will impair Yang at the superficial level; when it attacks the body internally, it will impair the internal Yang of organs. If Yang-Qi is impaired, and cannot warm and transform Qi, it will lead to Cold syndrome due to functional decline. If Cold impairs the surface of the body, the defensive Qi[4] will stagnate, leading to an aversion to cold and an inability to sweat. If Cold directly invades the Spleen and the Stomach, the Spleen-Yang will be impaired, leading to pain in the stomach and abdomen, vomiting, and diarrhoea.

Cold tends to coagulate: Cold can slow down the movements of matter and Qi. As temperature decreases, water can freeze, turning to ice. Qi, Blood, and Body Waters in the body flow continuously because they are constantly warmed and propelled by Yang-Qi.[5] If a pathogenic Cold obstructs Yang-Qi, then Qi, Blood, and

---

[4]The 'defensive Qi' — similar to the Western concept of the 'immune system' — is also called 'Wei Qi'.

[5]The warming Qi — which flows from Yang.

Body Waters cannot flow freely and will coagulate in the body's meridians, channels, and blood vessel: leading to blockage, pain, and vulnerability to other illness.

If Cold takes hold of internal organs, those internal organs will not function properly, impairing digestion, bowel movement, urination, breath, and so on. In turn, this can lead to difficulty breathing, wheezing, coughing, indigestion, diarrhoea, frequent passing of urine, menstrual problems, and pain. If Cold attacks the muscles and joints, Qi and Blood in the muscles and joints will atrophy, resulting in restriction of movement and localised pain in the muscles and joints. This can give rise to conditions such as arthritis.

Cold tends to contract: Cold pertains to Yin and tends to restrain the activity of Qi, leading to the contraction of muscles, tendons, and vessels. If Cold affects superficial parts of the body, pores will close, muscles will contract, and the defensive Qi (Wei Qi) cannot disperse leading to aversion to cold, inability to sweat, and goose pimples. If Cold invades limbs and joints, then tendons and vessels will become contracted, bringing on pain, headaches, and spasm of the limbs.

Heat (Fire)

Heat is also often named Fire.[6] In TCM, mild heat is a 'warm syndrome'; moderate heat is a 'heat syndrome';

---

[6] The two properties are intrinsically linked, though may be expressed differently under different conditions.

high heat is a 'fire syndrome'; and extreme heat is a 'toxic syndrome'.[7]

Heat is the predominant climatic factor in summer, particularly in southern China where pathogenic Heat (Fire) is of greatest concern. However, it can also be encountered in other seasons and other places.

Heat tends to flare up: Heat (Fire) pertains to Yang and tends to flare up.[8] This means that disease caused by the pathogenic Heat (Fire) tends to take place in the upper part of the body, or *moves* upwards at a fast pace. The symptoms are marked by high fever, aversion to heat, extreme thirst, a red face, and a fast and full pulse. Pathogenic Heat easily rises to disturb the mind, leading to insomnia, irritability, and even delirium. Like Wind, Heat syndromes also rapidly change from one state to another. Therefore, doctors must act fast and treat quickly.

Heat tends to consume Qi and impair body waters: Heat (Fire) pertains to Yang and tends to consume Yin-Qi. Heat from the sun can evaporate water in

---

[7] Differentiating these four degrees of Heat is complex. However, I teach my students a simple guide: check the coating of the tongue; if the coating on a patient's tongue is a little thin and yellow, it's a 'warm syndrome', thick and very yellow is a 'heat syndrome', a dark yellow and dry coating is a 'fire syndrome', and finally dark or even black, dry coating is a 'toxic syndrome'.

[8] Pun intended!

deserts, and similarly Heat affecting the body can also dry up the body's fluids.[9] If there is superabundant Heat, it will drive fluids out of the body in the form of sweat. As such, the diseases caused by pathogenic Heat are often accompanied by thirst, a dry throat and tongue, scanty and strong urine, a dry face, and dry skin. Due to overconsumption and the drying up of Body Waters, the Heat in the body can weaken Qi.[10]

Heat tends to produce Wind and disturb Blood: With the heat of summer come cyclones and typhoons. Similarly, if Heat invades the body, it can also cause Wind-related symptoms, such as convulsions. Heat will also cause a reckless movement of Blood outwards and upwards, and in the case of many 'Fire syndromes', we see red marks or bleeding on the skin, nose bleeds, and the coughing up of blood.

Heat tends to cause swelling and ulceration: Heat in nature causes expansion, so Heat in the body causes swelling. Parts of the body, swollen with stagnated Blood, can further putrefy — causing boils, which in turn can burst into an ulcer. In my clinic, I see many young people with acne, sometimes with boils and pus,

---

[9]For example, Heat can dry up saliva and cause thirst, or dry up Blood and cause dry skin.

[10]For example, profuse sweating due to an exuberance of Heat can impair the healthy Qi.

and I advise them to avoid Heat-promoting foods and drinks, as this will help their skin.

Another example of Heat syndrome is mouth ulcers: in TCM, frequent mouth ulcers are a typical sign of Heat syndrome.

Dryness

Dampness permeates the late summer in China, but in autumn this disappears, and the weather becomes cool and dry, with 'Dryness' predominant. TCM divides Dryness into 'Warm-Dryness' and 'Cool-Dryness' depending on the weather. Disease affected by the weather in early autumn is associated with Warm-Dryness syndrome, because there is still some remaining Summer-Heat; disease occurring due to the weather in late autumn is mostly associated with Cool-Dryness syndrome.

Dryness tends to impair the Lung: Dryness is prevalent in autumn and is associated with the Lung, impairing the organ when it invades the body. If Dryness impacts the Lungs, fluid in the lungs will be consumed and the organ's ability to eject toxins will be impaired in kind, leading to a dry cough with scanty phlegm, or sticky sputum that is difficult to cough up, leading to shortness of breath or chest pain. It follows that in clinical practice, TCM doctors see more patients suffer from lung or breathing problems in autumn.

Summer Heat

Summer-Heat is transformed from Heat and Fire in summer. It pertains to Yang, and in China usually peaks after the summer solstice and before the autumn solstice. Disease due to Summer-Heat follows as a direct result of exposure to hot weather, or due to the body's low adaptability to the summer environment.

Summer-Heat is extreme: Summer-Heat is the hottest of the year, so disease caused by Summer-Heat is usually marked by symptoms such as high fever, dysphoria, a reddish complexion, thirst, a full and fast pulse, and heat stroke. To prevent this, in the summer months, people across the Tropic of Cancer take siestas during the hottest part of the day — from Southern China to the Mediterranean.

Summer-Heat tends to rise and disperse: Summer-Heat tends to rise rapidly. If it invades the body, it can disturb the mind — leading to confusion, low mood, dizziness, and even episodes of fainting or sudden unconsciousness in severe cases. Summer-Heat induces sweating and reduces 'Body Waters' when it disperses, leading to thirst and dehydration, with dark, scanty urine. Following profuse sweating, Qi is lost, eventually bringing on shortness of breath and fatigue as a result of that deficiency.

Summer-Heat is often complicated by damp: In the hot summer season, Dampness often combines with Summer-Heat. Apart from the fever and thirst associated with Summer-Heat, symptoms that arise include vomiting, loose stools, and tiredness of the limbs.

Dampness

Dampness is an aetiological[11] concept unique to TCM. There is no equivalent in Western medicine so misunderstandings can occur, with matter lost in translation.

TCM identified two kinds of Dampness: internal and external. Internal Dampness refers to dysfunction of the Spleen and Kidney, which can result in toxins proliferating within a body's fluids. External Dampness arises from external environmental conditions.

External dampness is predominant in late summer but can be encountered in all seasons. Dampness permeates environments that are hot in late summer, and this combination can frequently cause disease. Exposing the body to the conditions of an excessively rainy or damp environment also results in Damp syndrome.

---

[11] Pertaining to medical diagnosis.

Dampness is heavy and turbid: Wet things are heavier than dry things, hence it follows Dampness is associated with a feeling of bloated heaviness in the head, limbs, and core. Water alone does not characterise Dampness; however, *stickiness* is an associated sign of Dampness, and manifests in the body as sticky saliva, mucus, stool, discharge from the ears and eyes, and turbid urine.[12]

Dampness tends to block Qi: Dampness is heavy and sticky, so therefore moves slowly, and tends to linger in the organs and meridians, inhibiting the flow of Qi and disrupting meridian activity. This leads to congestive symptoms, such as chest oppression, a feeling of fullness in the stomach, and difficulty with urination and constipation. On the other hand, Dampness pertains to Yin and tends to impair Yang-Qi. Thus, prolonged blockage of Qi by Dampness will prevent Yang-Qi from flowing smoothly, often causing a vicious cycle of exacerbating Dampness — a further accumulation of water — and the consequential decline of Yang. Among the Five Elements, Dampness pertains to Earth; as the organ principally associated with the Earth element, dampness actives most profoundly upon it. Damage rendered to the Spleen Yang leads to indigestion, bloating of the stomach, diarrhoea, and a swollen abdomen, ankles, or joints due to fluid build-up.

---

[12] That is to say, all excretions of the body become thicker and stickier under the influence of Damp.

Dampness is long lasting: The characteristics of Dampness usually affect people for a long time. This is because fluids constitute a majority of the body's mass, while Dampness toxifies those fluids by impairing the very organs that preserve flow and purity. Furthermore, we drink water every day in quantities that are not easy to gauge, and the food we eat also has high sugar and salt content, which both further the impact of Damp. When combined with the natural stickiness of Dampness, all of these attributes make Dampness a stubborn problem to treat.

Dampness tends to move downwards: Like water, Dampness sinks downwards. It therefore typically takes hold among the lower parts of the body first. The most common areas affected include the bowels, bladder, legs, and feet. The diseases caused by Dampness usually involve symptoms with a downwards tendency, such as discharge, diarrhoea, or a runny nose.

Diet

A poor diet is another common external cause of illness. Our diets can work against us in a manner of ways — most of which are related to the indulgence of extremes: too little or too much food; poor food quality; excessive deep-frying; excessive sugar, salt, fat, or meat; not drinking enough water; or overindulging in coffee, juices, supplements, or alcohol. The timing of meals is also pertinent, as is the manner of eating itself — eating too late at night, or too fast, or binge eating between periods of fasting. Even eating and talking too much at the same time is considered problematic in some schools of TCM!

In TCM, a great deal of emphasis is paid to the imitation of nature, as humans are a part of that nature. Above all, traditional Chinese doctors will advise their patients to obey the *rules of nature*: embracing them, rather than avoiding or, worse still, contradicting them.[13] Failing to follow these rules will result in unnecessary strain, stress, damage, or suffering. This applies to our diets too. We eat the foods the earth provides us with, at the right time and the right place. In an era of globalised production lines, mega-greenhouses, and factory farming, we can have all kinds of food in all seasons. Some may use this access to eat nothing but summer crops throughout a cold winter — watermelons, cucumbers, green salads, etc. — thinking it healthy, but TCM doctors would advise against such seasonal

---

[13] One of the many meanings held within the term 'Daoism' is its literal translation, i.e., 'the Way' or 'the Path'. A common image in Daoism is that of a great boulder blocking the path of running water. For the water to pass the rock, it needn't try to break the stone, or move it aside: or give up, and go back where it came from! The rules of nature instruct the water's 'way', which is around — and over time the boulder will become worn down, until eventually the pebble that is left flows with it. In this respect, following nature's 'Way' is both natural and easy; following the rules of nature in the way we live our lives is the 'Path' to health.

contradictions, which at length will cause imbalance in the body.[14]

Dietary Ailments

Poor quality food

Consuming poor-quality food is a sure-fire way to court illnesses of a wide variety. Quality in this case can refer to hygiene, to age, or to the presence of pesticides, radiation, pollution, or toxins.

Undereating

Meant both in terms of starvation and malnutrition — and of a limited *variety* of foods.[15]

I once treated a patient who encapsulated the importance of observing both these aspects. The patient in question, a young man with a skin condition (eczema) and hair loss, *did* consume an adequate amount of food: but that food he ate was limited to potato chips and chicken — and for many years. It was immediately evident to me, as it would be to any TCM practitioner, that this diet was the core component of his health troubles: where fried foods, like these potatoes, lead to excessive

---

[14]Further details on the relationship between diet, balance, and health are given in Chapter 7.

[15]Both the Chinese and Western dietary traditions agree in this sense; and the Western idiom that a 'colourful plate is a healthy plate' is echoed in Chinese thought.

Heat-syndrome — drying out and damaging skin, and where a lack of greater nutrient diversity is a classic cause of hair loss.

Excess

Obesity is one of the major causes of diabetes, heart problems, and a range of other, equally serious illnesses. Even for those who are not obese, craving or eating too much — or too much of one thing — can present health difficulties that in turn lead to illness.

Some food and drink — such as sugar, alcohol, and caffeinated fluids — can bring risk of addiction, if consumed in excess. However, even besides this extreme, excessive consumption of *any* food or drink can disrupt the body's Yin–Yang balance by introducing a disproportionate amount of one or more of the 'Six Evils' into the body.

Aseasonal and binge eating

Ancient Chinese thought holds that the Earth provides people with the 'right' foods at the 'right' time.[16] In

---

[16] This develops from the same core principle explored in Chapter 2: that the body is *of* and *from* nature: not separate to, but a part of, and extended from, the natural world. If this is true, it thereby follows that, under regular conditions, the provisions of a certain season would be fitting to and healthy for the body *in* those seasons — as it has evolved to fluctuate in harmony with the predictable fluctuating of environment, and the environment's harvestable food.

summer, we naturally harvest foods of a 'cooling' nature to combat the Summer-Heat, such as certain green vegetables and fruits. However, eating these same foods to excess in winter may further reduce the Summer-Heat that, in that season, is already in need of supplementation.

I have seen this dynamic play out many times among patients who have been programmed by Western pop-nutritionists into thinking that eating green vegetables and fruits to excess is *always* healthy. Those who wish to lose weight in winter frequently over-indulge in non-seasonal salads or juices. As a matter of fact, the more such patients exclusively eat such food, the more they will *develop* weight in the long term, because cold salads and juices will damage their Yang Qi in winter. This cycle internally develops their body's 'Cold', thereby slowing down their metabolism, with Yin further dominating Yang in the negative feedback loop that such a diet produces. Cold Qi cannot move Body Waters as efficiently, resulting in Dampness, and subsequent bloating and weight accumulation.

Mealtimes

It is especially common in modern life that meals are missed: resulting in individuals becoming disproportionately hungry, eating too late, and to excess. This behaviour can upend the body's natural rhythms, disrupting sleep and energy levels, which in turn impact mood, metabolism, and balance across the body's systems. This results in an increased vulnerability to illness across the board, with any existing vulnerability now made *that much more* susceptible to disease.

Diet and life cycle

TCM asserts that the diet of a new-born must be different from that of an old man. For women, for example, menstrual cycles, pregnancy, breastfeeding, and menopause all dictate certain dietary changes that should be recognised.[17] So, it is that each body's dietary needs will fluctuate — not just according to environmental conditions, or internal developments but also across time, according to age and state — such that resisting these changes presents a risk to health.

Other External Causes of Disease

Injury

Trauma:

a. **Direct damage**: Swelling, bruise, broken bones, and bleeding.

---

[17]Many of my Chinese friends come to the West and are shocked to find new mothers who have just delivered a baby eating ice cream or drinking cold water. Although this is clearly a cultural difference, it has been observed that women with these diets may develop problems later in life, such as arthritis or swollen legs (Cold-Damp conditions in TCM), problems which from my experience are far more common in the West than in China.

b. **Collateral damage**: Concussions, headache.
c. **Sequential damage**: Weakness, insomnia, indigestion, or even heart attack.
d. **Psychological damage**: Fear, depression, anxiety, phobia, etc.

Burns and scalds: Fire, hot water, steam, acids, scorching oil, and exposure to electric current and sunlight can cause burns and/or scalding. Heat is the common unifying factor here, with cooling methods the main treatment.

Frostbite: Caused by prolonged exposure to the cold. Cold freezes the blood and causes stasis of internal fluids, in turn leading to organ and tissue damage.

Bites by Insects, Beasts, and Other Animals

TCM specifically mentions the harm posed by insect stings and animal bites: which cause direct damage to the skin, muscles, tendon, or even bone. Some can further cause bleeding, festering, and poisoning due to the introduction of microorganisms or toxins into the body. The specific species that are warned against in Zhang Zhong Jing's seminal *Treatise on Febrile Diseases and Miscellaneous Diseases* are named on account of their presence in ancient China. However, the principal of this category of harm transcends geographic boundaries and should be guarded against in every environment.

Illness Caused by Medical Malpractice

A vast majority of medical professionals have chosen this career to help people, rather than to cause harm. Regardless of such good intentions, it is unfortunately true that misappropriated medical examinations and treatments can bear a degree of risk. Indeed, it has been claimed that, prior to the 20th century, Western medical doctors were responsible for *killing* more patients with their interventions than they saved![18]

X-rays and CT scans carry associated portions of radiation, while the excessive search for illness can carry a risk of psychological harm: with doubt and anxiety shifting to hypochondria if left unchecked. The overuse of antibiotics worldwide has for its part led to antibiotic-resistant 'superbugs', while the overenthusiastic prescription of opioids and sleeping tablets has led to addiction epidemics. Many medications elicit a wide range of destructive side effects, which is not to mention the unfortunate role that human error can play.

Even TCM, which practitioners are proud to consider safe and relatively non-invasive, can cause harm if used improperly. In acupuncture, inserting a needle too far

---

[18]This claim usually points its finger at medical practice up to the mass implementation of modern hygiene in the early 1900s, and to the mass rollout of penicillin in the 1940s: and the truth in it has been contested. Regardless, the argument stands that such medical interventions — no matter the intention behind them — can and do exacerbate illness when not properly implemented.

into certain points can result in tissue damage, while the incorrect application of certain herbal treatments can cause liver or kidney damage.

In another uncanny parallel to the Western tradition — in this case, to the well-known Hippocratic Oath — TCM masters will teach their students that the first priority of care should be to *do no harm*: with all therapeutic results a secondary concern.

Part Two: Internal Causes of Diseases

The internal causes of illnesses can be acquired or inherited. Acquired causes include lifestyle factors such as overeating or drinking, overwork, and lack of sleep. Inherited or constitutional vulnerabilities are called 'Jing Deficiencies', or 'essence' deficiency in TCM.[19] How strong our genetic 'Jing' is will be dependent on our parents' constitutions and the whole process of the pregnancy and birth. As an individual, you cannot change your inherited genetic 'Jing' — it's down to luck. But we can do something to mitigate a vulnerability if we know what it is: and by avoiding that vulnerability, we can help maintain health and prevent illness. A proactive preventive lifestyle is crucial to TCM.[20]

---

[19]Of course, TCM practitioners were not familiar with gene science or the structure of DNA — nevertheless, the tradition places great emphasis on family, and hereditary dynamics: especially in diagnosis and treatment.

[20]Chapter 7 explores preventative philosophy and its strategies: especially regarding the core principle of *balance*.

Lack of Inherited Jing

To pass a healthier 'Jing' on to offspring, TCM teaches that one must live a healthy lifestyle, behaving well, (avoiding alcohol, smoking, drugs, and an improper diet) and working to maintain a healthy body before conception. This way, and in turn, one's children will have the best chance at a healthy Jing. Avoiding these rules risks producing offspring that bears a 'deficient' Jing — one that is weaker in its constitution: more vulnerable to internal and congenital disease.

Stress

Long-term mental stress is a major cause of illness. Stress consumes Qi and Blood in equal measure, taxing the Liver Qi and Blood especially. This stretches liver function to its limits, leading in time to liver-related disease.

Work

Whether it be physical or mental (or both), excessive hours, related exhaustion, strain, and physical injury naturally lead to illness. In the modern world, expectations are high: employees expect greater and greater productivity of *themselves*, while employers expect greater productivity of their labour. This cycle is active near universally, despite the incredible wealth that society has already achieved. This kind of greed can cause Heart and Spleen problems. In TCM, as in the Buddhism that informed it, contentment and gratitude are taught as a way of interrupting and shattering this unhealthy negative feedback loop: reorienting us towards healthier expectations — and a happier life.

Lack of Work

To the opposite extreme, too much rest — or a lack of work — presents its own disruptive force. Daily work is natural and helps energise the flow of Qi and Blood: strengthening body and mind.

Emotions

Of all internal causes, emotion (or, rather, emotional excess) is the most common cause for chronic and serious disease. In TCM, we address this as problem of the 'Seven Emotions': joy, anger, anxiety, worry, grief, terror, and fear. These are emotions we all experience. Provided they are not overly powerful, they contribute to a normal part of a healthy life and will not in themselves cause illness. However, if control should slip, these forces can and will become toxic. Across the tens of thousands of patients I have seen in my time practicing TCM, I am confident in saying that the most common cause of illness is our own emotions.

Why do emotions play such important roles in the causation of our illnesses? TCM answers this question by advocating a kind of mind–body dualism.[21] It holds that

---

[21] Fittingly, this is *also* a Cartesian perspective!

human bodies are unique in this world, constructed as they are of two parts: structural and functional. The structural part is the chassis, or 'machine', and the functional parts are the controls. The machine can be defective: but most of those that survive past birth have usually proved themselves rigid enough. However, the controls are another matter entirely — and developing them in a healthy or constructive manner can be extraordinarily difficult. In TCM, these 'controls' refer to our neurological functions, but just as much to our knowledge, wisdom, experiences, ideologies, will power, and discipline.

Not all controls are inherited, nor are all spontaneous: each body must learn to develop its own controls *inside itself*. The consequences of 'defective' controls do not articulate themselves before or during birth — when the structure is tested — but in the years after when 'health' is a concern. By the time bodies are driven by their controls to eat or drink themselves to death, or smoke and use drugs, or fight uncontrollably, doctors can do very little beyond helping the acute symptoms.

In TCM, emotions are associated with corresponding physical organs. Should disease take root in a physical organ, that disruption will manifest itself in the state of the corresponding emotion.[22] In TCM, the Liver is

---

[22] Consider the typical dualism of Yin Yang, as illustrated in Figure 4 of Chapter 2. As the Mind/Body pair exists in opposition and complementation to one another, the two parts

linked with anger[23]; a patient suffering from disease of the liver (hepatitis, for example, or liver cancer) will become vulnerable to outbursts of anger, or short temperedness. In the Tradition, if a person has too much liver 'Heat', he may have a red face and bloodshot eyes; eager to fight, a doctor would diagnose him with 'Liver Fire' ('Gan Huo').

Seven Emotions

Emotions are natural functions, and fluctuations within a certain degree are completely normal and do not cause illness. However, an overly intense or prolonged emotional response will surpass the regulative adaptability of the human body, resulting in the disruption of internal Qi. In these circumstances the balance between Qi and Blood — Yin and Yang — is broken, resulting in illness.

Unlike the aforementioned Six Evils that penetrate from without to cause disease within, the Seven Emotions cause damage to the inner body, particularly to its Qi. As Qi powers the functions of our organs, damage to Qi leads to organ dysfunction, such as low energy, slow movements of the bowels, lack of urination control, low libido, and sensations of pain. At the

---

interlink — revealing their interdependency. Change in the matter/form of one part is necessarily reflected through equal, opposite, and parallel change in the other.

[23] Healthy liver functioning provides for a 'long fuse', as it were!

early stages, tangible change is gradual, but if Qi is disturbed for prolonged periods, then masses, lumps, or tumours can arise.

The Seven Emotions are closely linked to the Five Elements — as explored in Chapter 2,[24] each of Five Elements' organs is dominated by one kind of emotion:

- Heart — joy
- Liver — anger
- Spleen — contemplation
- Lung — grief
- Kidney — terror

The emotion and organ mutually direct one another. If the Liver Qi is made sick, the patient will express anger or aggression, while in a state of flow, the same patient will express serenity.

Beyond the Five Elements, there are two additional emotions: anxiety (associated with both Lung and Liver) and fear (associated with the Heart).

---

[24] These lists of 'Five X' and 'Seven Y' may be overwhelming at first: however, the numbers themselves have great significance in Chinese culture, and appreciating this significance is important to fully comprehending TCM. For instance, both Five and Seven appear frequently in Chinese folk tales — drawn from the same era that gave rise to TCM. In one, a dead man's spirit lingers on earth for seven days after his death.

1. *Excessive joy*: Joy is the emotion of the Heart. Joy and happiness stimulate a smoother flow of Heart Qi and Blood. Excessive joy may result in the disruption of Heart Qi, so that the Shen ('mind') is inhibited, leading to the absence of mind, and mania. Joy is usually a good thing, but as the Yin/Yang model illustrates, any movement to extremes results in collapse: a 'good' feeling can thereby inflate into its opposite, and collapse into 'bad'.

2. *Excessive anger*: Anger is related to the Liver. Excessive anger can cause Liver Qi imbalance, leading to a superabundance of and hyperactivity of Liver-Yang, itself leading to flare-ups of violent rage. This incurs headaches, bad mood, sudden dizziness, loss of consciousness, paralysis, distorted facial expression, and can even result in a stroke. Tracking from the body: should a patient suffer from liver disease, they will be quick to anger.

3. *Excessive contemplation*: Contemplation is related to the Spleen. Excessive contemplation will stagnate Spleen-Qi and affect transportation and transformation, leading to gastric and abdominal distension and fullness, poor appetite, anorexia, and loose stools. Prolonged indulgence in contemplation consumes Yin and Blood and deprives the Heart-spirit of nourishment, often bringing on palpitations, amnesia, insomnia, and dreaminess.

4. *Excessive grief or sadness*: Excessive grief can exhaust Qi. Grief is dominated by the Lung Qi.

Excessive grief exhausts Lung-Qi. Prolonged and excessive grief affects the ability of the Lung to purify, descend, disperse, and distribute matter and fluid. This results in failure of distribution of nutrient (Ying) Qi and defensive (Wei) Qi: leading to dizziness, fatigue, and dispiritedness.

5. *Excessive terror*: Excessive terror can drive Qi to move downwards. Terror is dominated by the Kidney. Sudden terror drives the Kidney-Qi to move downwards, and as it becomes dislodged this leads to incontinence, atrophy of the bones, and seminal emission: due to failure of the Kidney to store Essence (Jing).[25]

6. *Excessive anxiety*: Anxiety is related to the Liver and the Lung. Excessive anxiety may impair the Lung and the Liver. Anxiety usually inhibits Qi and leads to depression of Lung-Qi, and/or stagnation of Liver-Qi. The depression of Lung-Qi causes difficulty breathing, while stagnation of Liver-Qi leads to hypochondriac distension and fullness or pain.

7. *Excessive fear*: Fear and terror are similar emotions, but they have a different effect on Qi. Terror, dominated by the Kidney, drives Qi to move downwards; fear, originating from the Heart, disturbs the activity of Heart-Qi. So, with excessive fear, the main response is a disorder of Heart-Qi, derangement of the mind,

---

[25] A prolonged state of terror may lead to various illnesses due to failure of the Kidney-Qi and Yang to elevate and defend the body.

indecision, and bewilderment. Disorder of the activity of the Heart-Qi damages the harmony between Qi and Blood, weakening the defensive Qi, resulting in greater vulnerability to pathogenic factors and disease.

Lack of Sexual Discipline

In TCM, normal sexual activity is helpful for the flow of Qi and the regulation of Yin and Yang. It has been argued by TCM practitioners that avoiding sexual activity can lead to illness. However, the more pressing issues today are those surrounding excessive sex and excessive desire. This will consume too much Qi and the Essence (Jing) of the Kidney, leading to early senility with symptoms of dizziness, tinnitus, dispiritedness, impotence or low libido, and memory problems.

But this demands specificity! What is excessive? How much is too much? Of course, there is no definite or absolute figure, but one catered for and relative to each individual, depending on age, constitution, health, and so on: even the season and one's workload hold relevance here!

Age: Only mature people can have sex: children and underage people cannot and should not. When one is still maturing into adulthood, he/she needs all their Essence (Jing) for the body and its development. In the tradition, both eggs and sperm are a part of this Jing. Sex will release this aspect of Essence, and if one is not yet mature, the Jing will be excessively taxed, leading to weakness of the Kidney, of the defensive Qi, and, in later life, to premature aging. Once mature, a healthy frequency of sex is dependent on age, with a gradual decline in necessary frequency as one grows older being quite natural.

Basic health: Basic health is of course a very important factor for the appropriate frequency of sex. For those people who have Kidney or Heart issues, less sex is ideal.

Workload: When one works hard and tires out, one should rest — to recuperate strength and energy. Forcing sex at such times incurs a double tax upon the body — further weakening it.

Seasons: We all know that animals have their mating seasons. Humans are a part of nature too, and a seasonal change in sexual activity should be admitted. TCM encourages us to have less sex in autumn and winter seasons — when Cold, Wind, and Dryness permeate.

Excessive sexual thoughts: Excessive sexual thoughts, such as an addiction to pornography, will weaken your Jing. I once treated a 30-year-old male patient who suffered from dizziness, tiredness, insomnia, and impotency. Through our discussions, I learned that he started watching pornographic films at the age of 10 and had become addicted to them. In his 20s, he could not have normal sex, and the sensation of impotency worsened. All his other symptoms, from the dizziness to the tiredness and the insomnia, derived ultimately from a Kidney Jing deficiency, stemming from this addiction.

Secondary Causes of Diseases

The following details are not *root* factors of disease, but are nevertheless important to note, as their presence and production within the body can lead to secondary health issues.

Phlegm: In TCM, Phlegm is considered a thick and functionless Body Fluid. When it is produced, it should be discharged from the body. If it stays in the body, it occupies space, blocking the meridians and complicating diseases, leading to lumps or swelling. If Phlegm is moving in a meridian, we call this 'Wind-Phlegm', and this is the major cause of stroke and vertigo.

Stale Blood: If Blood is not moving properly within the organs or body, and not resident in the Liver, then it is considered 'stale' Blood. When Blood runs out of the body's meridians entirely — then it is 'dead' Blood. Such Blood has no function and is therefore useless and harmful to the body. If it overstays its welcome, it will block the movement of Qi and Blood, resulting in further impairment. This 'stale' Blood can cause bleeding, lumps, dark discolouration of the skin, and sharp pain.

Retained food: If food is left undigested, or not digested properly, and remains in the intestines, it can become toxic. When the bowels are blocked, then digestive functions become severely disturbed. The body finds it difficult to get the nutrition it needs, instead absorbing toxins from the undigested food. Qi deficiency and Blood deficiency are common consequences, which is especially problematic for young children, whose growth may be restricted as a result.

Chapter 4

Mechanisms of Illness

Having established the traditional understandings of *cause*, let us now turn to the *method* by which illness can take hold. How is it that these internal and external dynamics manifest as disease? Would all patients become sick, should they encounter the same internal/external cause? Would that sickness take the same form in one patient as another? Would they be equally severe? Will it develop consistently, and would the same treatments produce the same effects?

In answering these questions, and exploring the mechanisms through which disease takes root, we will encounter the dialectical processes that TCM observes within the body. However, before we can, we must first make clear exactly what 'illness' is.

Part One: What is Illness?

What does Traditional Chinese Medicine consider 'illness'? The concept is continuous with disease, sickness, morbidity, and disorder, and as in Western medicine, these terms are often used interchangeably. Yet, it would be a mistake to assume that TCM regards illness identically to the Western tradition.

In Western medicine, the diagnosis of an illness is a black and white affair. In its terms, diseases such as cancers, infections, hypertension, osteoporosis, arthritis, and psoriasis are reducible to a clear clinical symptoms and signs, backed by hard, repeatable evidence provided by clinical test data.

Diagnosis in Western medicine is a binary matter: one may be ill or not ill. If the body is sick, it is sick with a specific, known, and demonstrably measurable sickness. To the contrary, diagnosis in TCM is closer to an art. Illness in TCM is not a clear, measurable quantity. As we explored in Chapter 2, the 'reason' that informs TCM is drawn not from the scientific method but theological, social, and cultural ethics. Such reason comprises the vague space between 'good' and 'bad', 'health' and 'sickness' — as in nature, where states of nuance exist in all things.

As we all know, nobody 'gets' cancer, osteoporosis, hypertension, arthritis, or psoriasis overnight, or in a flash. All illnesses — even infections — take time to form and develop. Before a diagnosis can be made, there will invariably be a period of time during which no symptoms or signs are present. When the earliest symptoms do present, they generally take hold subtly, such that patients and doctors often miss the early signs of an illness, when timely treatment would be most effective.

Modern medicine has made significant process in bridging this gap and enabling the early detection of illness. MRI, CT, PET scans, DNA testing, and a host of other diagnostic techniques have enabled the application of early treatments — through which many lives have been saved. Yet, even these tools rely upon the presence of symptoms to direct their application. Once symptoms have expressed themselves to such a degree that diagnosis is attempted, the illness has already taken hold: thus, regardless of how early an illness is diagnosed, it is often too late to apply the 'ideal' early-stage intervention. This is a core and inherent contradiction in Western, 'treatment'-oriented medicine: the emphasis on addressing a specific illness, once it has been observed, positions the doctor forever 'behind' the development of that illness.

One might observe that the natural solution is a system in which illnesses are addressed *before* they take hold, and symptoms show. That is where TCM directs its focus. The concept of treating an illness before it starts is essential to our practice. Therefore, TCM's definition of illness contains not only the clinical realities of symptoms and signs but also the diseased *conditions* of life: and the wayward trajectory of a patient's health.

There is a folk story in China about the king of a small province, thousands of years ago. One day, this king was approached by the court doctor, who said to him 'Your Majesty, I have observed you these past months, and I believe you are sick, and are in need of my treatments'. At this, the king laughed: and all his ministers laughed with him. Mocking the doctor, the king said, 'I feel fine! Doctors are nothing but attention seekers; this one exaggerates my health issues to try and win my favour'. Several months passed and the doctor met with the king again — immediately telling him that his illness had worsened. It was now an issue of vital importance, in need of urgent care. To this, the king laughed once again — dismissing the doctor with the same confident air.

The third time the doctor met the king at the gates of palace. This time the doctor said nothing but ran at the sight of him. The king was puzzled and sent his attendants to call the doctor back to the palace to explain himself: but the doctor refused. He explained the king was on the verge of a dire illness — and that it was too late for any treatments to take effect. 'If I am in the palace when the king dies', he said, 'I will be blamed as a useless doctor, and it will mean my head'. Indeed, a few weeks later, the king fell ill, dying in the days that followed. When asked how he had known, the doctor explained that the first time he had seen the king he had recognised a sickness at the superficial level — one that was easily treated with modifications in lifestyle and diet. The second time, that sickness had developed — penetrating the organs. While radical, the doctor's herb and acupuncture methods would still have treated the king. But by the third time, the sickness has penetrated the 'Gao Huang' — the core of a man, deep in his chest, — which no doctor could treat once diseased.

Of course, the 'moral' of this story illustrates the importance of addressing an illness in its time. But the story also speaks to the *definition* of illness in TCM. Thousands of years old, stories like this one informed the tradition as it developed, and the perspective it formed is one that teaches illness as a consequence of life as it is (mis)led: not a singular episode, but a state, out of which we can be guided — given timely intervention.

In TCM, a healthy body or person is one that is simply well balanced in all respects.[1] Inwardly, there is balance among all parts of the body: the Jing; Qi and Shen; Qi and Blood; Yin and Yang; and all the organs, tissues, and meridians. Outwardly, there is balance between the body and seasons, geolocations, food and diet, work, and leisure, as well as harmony with family and society.

---

[1]Chapter 7 explores the relationship between Balance and Health.

Part Two: The Mechanisms of Illness in TCM

Zhen Qi

How can the balance of the body be broken? Why is it that, when faced with the same forces, some people become ill where others do not?

In TCM, we believe this depends on the body's ability to defend itself against external or internal causes of disease, known as 'Evil Qi'. This ability to defend stems from our 'vital energy', called the 'Zhen Qi'. Zhen Qi in Chinese translates to 'Correct Qi', referring to all natural bodily aspects, such as Jing, Qi (all kinds), and Shen.

As a rough analogy, imagine the body as a house, occupied by Zhen Qi, the 'good matter'. The 'bad matter', such as viruses, cannot get in because the house is already full: there is no room! This is an especially important principle in TCM — cultivating the Zhen Qi, rather than tackling the Evil Qi, in order to treat an illness (forcing it out of the house) or to prevent it from developing in the first place (forbid it from entering).[2]

Western doctors might understand Zhen Qi as *roughly* equivalent to the concept of the immune system, and

---

[2]In Chinese society, people will speak colloquially about the 'best', 'good', and 'average' TCM doctors — the average ones treat while the best ones prevent!

it's easy to grasp how infectious diseases may arise from a weak immune system. However, in TCM, we also consider many other problems, such as insomnia or depression, to be related to a weakness of Zhen Qi.[3] Regardless, I cannot say that there is a one-to-one equivalence between the TCM concept of Zhen Qi and the Western concept of the immune system. From clinical practice, what we *can* say is that health breeds health, and that health defends against sickness.[4]

TCM often conceives of the development of illness in terms of a great battle between Zhen Qi, our 'vital energy', and Evil Qi, the external and internal causes of disease. If Zhen Qi is stronger than Evil Qi, illness can be prevented or minimised. On the other hand, if Zhen Qi is weaker than Evil Qi, illness will develop, or increase in severity.

Recognising Illness — Administering Treatment

By comparing Western and Traditional Chinese Medicines in this way, a broad distinction can be made whereby the former recognises illness once present, or else does not, while TCM considers 'illness' and

---

[3] In the scientific community, there is indeed growing evidence that the immune system may be related to a myriad of problems, including depression, but this is still a relatively new area of scientific research.

[4] Thus, supporting the concept of Zhen Qi. For example, a positive mentality leads to less 'room' for negative thoughts, leaving a lower chance of developing illness or depression.

'health' existing upon a live and dynamic continuum. When health is associated with balance and illness imbalance, there exist varying states of balance and imbalance between those extremes. When a body exists in the 'grey area' between extremes, then the symptoms of illness may not be severe enough to prompt immediate recognition or diagnosis by Western means: nevertheless, if the imbalance is neglected, then that sickness will likely develop.

In TCM, we use the term 'Wei Bing', which can be translated into 'not yet ill', to describe this 'grey area'. The tradition emphasises the importance of dealing with these 'grey area' states in order to strengthen the Qi and Wei Qi: bringing the body back to health and preventing the articulation of disease. When concerned with Wei Bing, it is of course difficult to distinguish the precise Evil Qi at work, and to pinpoint a clear diagnosis.[5] As a result, TCM specialists will use more generic terms (such as 'weakness' and 'deficiency') as catch-all phrases that cover the unknowns within 'grey area' states.[6]

---

[5] If symptoms have not yet developed to severity, then the signs a doctor needs to interpret the nature of imbalance will not show.

[6] To Western ears, the imprecision of such terms may suggest an unscientific method. On the contrary, the use of these terms is not emblematic of pseudo-scientific 'Cold Reading' or similar — but rather reflects the challenge of limited evidence. While Western medicine would not diagnose at all, TCM holds that responsible action can still be taken in the 'grey area' — though the expression of limited evidence is held in the language used.

So, why and how does this state of 'imbalance', or illness, arise?

This might follow an imbalance between the body's Zhen Qi and external factors (the aforementioned 'Evil Qi') such as Heat, Cold, or Dampness. Or, this might follow an imbalance of internal factors — with disruption within the unified whole of the body's Five Elements: (1) Yin/Yang, (2) the organs, and (3) Jing, (4) Qi, and (5) Shen. A problem with one element will lead to an imbalance across the body, giving rise to consequential effects elsewhere.

Imbalance also arises due to unnatural changes and distorted life cycles, such as premature or overdue birth, or menstrual cycles that are too light or heavy. Despite this, it is important to note that the slow accumulation of wear and tear — mounting the imbalances they deliver upon the body *as such* — is a natural aspect of the human experience. While TCM observes the relationship between imbalance and illness, it does propose to 'solve' the question of mortality! Its practice is built out of nature, just as the body arises *from* nature: and as eventual illness and death is a natural process, so too is TCM limited to treating only the *unnatural* imbalance brought on by internal and external causes.[7]

---

[7] The question of *when* death is 'natural' is one of ethics, not practice — and while fascinating, the philosophies of medical ethics do not sit within the scope of this book. The sharp rise of geriatric medicine in the West reveals those societies' unresolved

Unlike Western medicine, TCM does not view illness — or the human body — as a purely mechanical process. Of course, it is tempting to do so: when we eat more food, we gain weight; when we regularly exercise, we grow stronger; when we sleep well, we awaken revitalised.

And yet — as a consequence of observations made over the course of millennia — TCM appreciates that the body does not always express a logical and proportional response to behaviour. When eating more food, circumstances might arise in which we lose weight! Exercising more frequently might cause injury, weakening the body, while excessive sleep frequently results in sluggishness and lethargy. TCM asserts that the human is composed of a multitude of interrelated, interdependent forces. The clear mechanical logic that applies to car repair does not necessarily hold for human patients.

TCM doctors are not mechanics. They cannot approach a body with a schematic — jumping *with* knowledge *to* solution. The work starts in the study of a body's Five Elements — to know, then understand,

---

approaches to this question, and debate surrounding it continues in TCM just as it does in the West. Nevertheless, while few doctors of *either* tradition would argue that there is a precise point at which treatment should be suspended, it is demonstrably true that age brings imbalance, which in turn brings illness and death: which is the point of our observation here.

and only *then* treat. Having investigated the balance between elements — under the conditions of potential Evil Qis — treatments are recommended not by rote but as response: and the mechanics at work may vary as much as we find that bodies and environments do.

Chapter 5
Diagnosis

Like that in Western medicine, diagnostic examination in TCM involves the application of methodologies in the pursuit of information on a patient's clinical state. Doctors will apply medical theory, knowledge, and experience when analysing this information, with the goal of ultimately identifying the core illness.

Here, I present two diagnostic cases, serving as an aperture through which we may explore this process, and from which we may derive the essential principals of diagnosis in the tradition.

Part One: Case Studies

Case 1

I met Mrs. P some years ago. An 80-year-old woman, she initially presented with shingles on her back, which she had suffered from for several weeks. Before contacting me she had consulted her GP, who had diagnosed the condition and prescribed painkillers and a palliative cream. Her core symptoms were the blisters on her back, accompanied by a severe and painful burning sensation. The GP gave her some cream and painkillers.

After one week of using the medications, the blisters on her back had begun to heal, but the pain had worsened. She could not sleep, and the painkillers had no effect.

At the same time, an odd change occurred: her tongue (or rather, the coating of her tongue) became black, as if she had smoked for many years. This new symptom caused her to panic, and she visited the GP again to ask after this development. After discovering that she had never smoked, the doctor admitted to not knowing — and left the matter there.

As the pain got worse, Mrs. P's daughter found me — and we soon arranged for an appointment. She explained that her pain was *burning* in quality, and that she had experienced constipation as a side effect of the painkillers, which in turn had done nothing to alleviate that pain. She also reported hot flushes, remitting thirsts, and had a red tongue with a dry, thick black coating, accompanied by a rapid pulse. Her urine was of a strong yellow colour.

From the symptoms and signs, I concluded Mrs. P suffered from a Heat distortion. I explained to her that the shingles infection was a point at which external Heat was invading her body, causing the skin blisters and the pain.

The cream she used to heal the blisters seemed effective, but this was a mistake. It sealed Heat inside the body, and there was no way for this to dissipate. Her constipation, brought on by the painkillers, blocked the escape of Heat from the body yet further. Her pain thereby got worse, despite the skin at first getting better. This trapped Heat in the body flared up, rising to the upper part of the body coating her tongue with a burnt ash black.

Once diagnosed, I prescribed some cooling and purging herbs to clear that Heat from her body, and applied acupuncture to various points of the Large Intestine channel, to further diffuse the internal Heat. I explained that the only side effect would follow from the herbs combined with the acupuncture treatment, which may induce temporary diarrhoea as the trapped Heat was released. She agreed, eager to progress with the treatment.

After a few days of treatment with mild diarrhoea, her pain remitted and later dissolved completely over the course of several weeks. Her tongue even returned to its original hue!

This case demonstrates the activity of external Heat in TCM. From the manifestation of Mrs. P's symptoms (especially the burning pain — though the black tongue, rapid pulse, and constipation further support it), a causal Heat syndrome can be clearly identified. Regardless of the infection that may be present — be it viral, fungal, or bacterial — in TCM, any one of these will deliver the 'Evil Qi' of external Heat, thereby causing bodily disruption and pain as a result of subsequent imbalance.[1] Once excessive external Heat has been diagnosed, the priority of treatment should be to clear the Heat that has accumulated inside the body.

There are a number of the ways to eliminate Heat from the body. Sweating, urinating, and purging are some, and in a healthy body these occur as a natural response. In the case of Mrs. P, the black coating was a key sign indicating the severity of the Heat, which had disrupted the body's natural ability to disperse the excess. Purging the Heat through the bowels with herbs and acupuncture suited her case well and fortunately this route took immediate effect.

---

[1] In its attempt to explain the core reason and logic of TCM to a Western reader, this book should dispel the untrue notion that the Chinese Tradition actively rejects Western scientific notions. Note that in this case, as in many others, the TCM diagnosis and treatment do not directly contradict the Western approach. Indeed, both the TCM and Western diagnoses agree upon the scientific cause of the sickness (namely, microbiotic infection, potentially enabled by a vulnerable immune system), while it is merely the treatment that differs — each, according to its school.

While still essentially non-invasive,[2] purging therapy is not a common choice for an 80-year-old patient in TCM. Nevertheless, given the urgency brought on by the pain Mrs. P was enduring, I judged this to be the safest course of action. While the cream and painkiller approach sought to address her symptoms, the purging of the Heat is what TCM doctors refer to as 'Root Treatment'[3]: realising a deeper, more sustained recovery.

Case 2

Some time ago I met J, a 2-year-old boy whose parents had brought him to me following a severe bout of eczema. J's skin was extremely red and inflamed, marked in many areas by scratch wounds brought on by the itchiness. He cried each night, could not sleep, and would not cover his body with the duvet for fear of the sensation. J's parents had taken him to a range of

---

[2] For a vulnerable or elderly patient, *both* schools of medicine will concern themselves with minimalising the potential harm that may be caused by a treatment plan. Nevertheless, as explored in Chapters 2 and 3, it is generally true to say that TCM treatments are less invasive than their Western counterparts. In this case, the antiseptic cream and codeine risked harm to the patient (a risk that was in part realised); the herbal purging, while difficult in its own respect, merely induced a natural bodily function — incurring less risk to the patient — as is typical of TCM.

[3] See Glossary. A 'Root Treatment' is any treatment that seeks to tackle the core/essential cause of an illness — reducing the symptoms by addressing their source.

dermatologists, who had all treated the eczema with various steroid creams. These induced a short-term relief whenever the cream was applied, but the condition did not get better, and the parents were desperate to solve the underlying problem.

Examining the boy revealed his skin to be red, dry, and hot to the touch, while his tongue was a deep red — with the tissue itself, cracked. I explained to the parents the boy had too much Heat in his body, and that this followed from a weakness in his kidney. The weakness in the kidney resulted in a disruption of Body Waters, which could not cool the body down as they otherwise would, and so, could not balance or reduce this Heat. The excess Heat caused the painfully inflamed skin — and his red cracked tongue. I prescribed a range of herbs and insisted on a set of dietary amendments: for example, avoiding deep-fried foods and citrus and spice, as TCM considers these 'Hot' in nature. Following this treatment, the boy's pain subsided, and his eczema was almost entirely healed. The parents, however, were concerned about what I had said regarding the boy's kidneys and went to see a Western doctor to conduct kidney tests. These test results all came back normal, and they were advised that there was nothing wrong: and the family stopped seeing me as a result.

However, 5 years on, the boy suddenly developed problems urinating, and hospital scans showed that one of the boy's kidneys had shrunk to the size of a walnut. His doctor could offer no explanation. Having remembered what I had said years earlier, the parents returned to me. Unfortunately, I could not reverse the physical changes to his kidney at this point but advised that further care should be taken for the other kidney.

This is a typical case of paediatric eczema. The Western dermatologists' diagnoses and treatments were all correct, as evidenced by the short-term results they secured. However, these results could not last, because the steroid creams only provided a superficial, symptom-oriented solution.

As explored in Chapter 2, the Yin–Yang balance of Heat and Cold is of primal importance to bodily health. In the case of J, the balance had tipped, with excessive Yang dominating insufficient Yin — with too much Heat and not enough Cooling: the balances were tilted to Heat and Yang. The consequence of this imbalance manifested in the skin, with dry red rashes, itchiness, and excessive internal Heat resulting in restlessness.

Why did J have too much Yang, or Heat, inside the body? Common causes of excessive Heat include an imbalanced diet, or too much alcohol (appropriately named 'fire water' in some languages), smoking, or too much emotional stress. However, J was a young child, so it is hard to imagine him turning to whiskey and cigarettes after a long day at the office! However, *as* a child, he was developing fast — with the fast metabolism that causes children to eat more relative to their size — and to become hungry more quickly, and more often. Just as feeding an engine extra coal raises the temperature of the flame, the speed of the pistons, and the volume of hot waste — the faster metabolic rate of youth raises conditions of Heat within the body.

On the other hand, all organs of children are still immature — making them more susceptible to imbalance — and this is especially true of the kidneys. Why the kidneys especially? Proportionally, children have more water in the body than adults — so their kidneys must work harder to maintain the balance of the water within the body. If children do not drink enough water (and quite often they forget!), then they quickly become victim to excessive Heat.

On top of these reasons, what made me so certain about this boy's potential kidney problems was the cracking on the tongue. Should children express Heat at such a young age, it will commonly express itself as thirst, as a red face and skin, or through dark yellow urine and restlessness. A cracking tongue, on the other hand, reflects a disorder in the organ itself, corresponding to a deep dehydration which necessarily involves the actual kidney — and not just daily environmental changes.

Such fundamental changes in the body's organs take time. The eczema was an early symptom of Heat syndrome, which only later manifested in the kidney's structural change after years had passed — during which time the body's Yang/Heat imbalance had dominated. Additional dietary issues, stress, or pressure during this time would have further contributed to the shrinkage. Unfortunately, this unaddressed cycle of Heat syndrome had caused irreversible harm in J, though I subsequently worked with the patient's parents to provide dietary and lifestyle recommendations that would limit the damage rendered by this change.

Part Two: Diagnostic Methods and Clinical Information

Four Methods

TCM diagnosis consists of four methods:

1. Inspection,
2. Auscultation[4] and Olfaction,[5]
3. Interrogation,
4. Palpation[6] and Pulse-Taking.

The following examination provides a broad outline of these methods: for technical analysis, I would recommend referring to a TCM diagnostics textbook.[7]

---

[4] See Glossary, listening to the heart.
[5] See Glossary, reviewing the sense of smell.
[6] See Glossary, inspecting the body through touch.
[7] See Bibliography, *The Essential Book of Traditional Chinese Medicine* by Liu Yanchi, Columbia University Press, New York, 1988. And *Diagnostics of Traditional Chinese Medicine* by Wang Lufen and Zuo Yanfu, compiled by Nanjing University of Traditional Chinese Medicine, Shanghai Pujiang Education Press, 2002.

1. Inspection

Inspection begins the moment the patient walks into the consulting room. A doctor considers the way the patient walks and talks, considers their movements, their complexion, and their manner. We then transition from this more general inspection to a more specific and localised one, as the appointment progresses. If required, we will even inspect samples of urine, stool, phlegm, and other excretions.

Something unique to TCM is its emphasis on inspecting the eyes and tongue, and of the meaning of this data in relation to diagnosis. In the Tradition, it is often said that 'the eyes are the windows of the spirit' and 'the tongue is the window to the body'. Accordingly, we put stock in our inspections of the eyes and tongue when determining the psychological and bodily health of the patient, respectively.

During every consultation, a TCM doctor must examine the patient's tongue. Together with checking a patient's pulse, this is considered one of the most important diagnostic techniques — because it provides a key insight into the whole body. So, why is it that the tongue functions as a 'window to the body'?

Firstly, we consider the tongue as an 'organ' of the internal body as it exists under the same internal conditions, and yet is the only such inner organ that is easy to access and inspect from the outside. Further, in TCM theory, the tongue is connected to all the organs in the body through intangible meridians — and it is especially linked directly to the Heart (the 'emperor organ'). In reflecting the status of the inner body, and through its meridian connections, the tongue is a sensitive and early indicator of bodily change. This change can be positive — as the successful transition in Case 1 demonstrated — or negative, as an illness develops and the condition of the tongue worsens.

Some experienced TCM doctors can pick up minute changes on the tongue that contribute to an early diagnosis — or predict a future illness that has yet to take hold: even if the patient does not yet have other tangible signs, symptoms, or test results. Like the ability of some animals to sense an earthquake, hurricane, or volcanic eruption long before it happens, we believe that all illnesses will affect the body in a ripple effect and transmit a kind of signal — albeit a weak signal — which skilled TCM practitioners can often detect in the tongue first.[8]

Secondly, a tongue is a useful 'window to the body' because it has a consistent appearance across race, age,

---

[8]I have a patient who I advise not to drink alcohol as a result of her internal conditions. She normally follows my advice well — though occasionally drinks a little on Friday nights, with her appointments following on Saturday mornings. When I inspect her tongue, this reveals that she has had a drink during the week, and she often says, "Damn! You always pick up my only night of drinking!"

and gender. While people can and do change their outward appearance, that of the tongue is less easy to alter. Brushing or scratching your tongue, for example, will only give rise to short-term changes.[9]

When a TCM doctor inspects the tongue, they will examine the body (form), the coating, and the functioning.

In terms of the tongue's body (form), a doctor will inspect the size, shape, colour, thickness, and moistness of the tongue, and whether these vary across parts. They will also check for unusual marks on the tongue, such as spots, cracks, cuts, and scars, noting their colour, size, position, and distribution. For example, pink is the healthiest colour for the tongue: a red tongue usually suggests excessive Heat in the body. If the redness only appears on the tip of the tongue, this indicates Heat in the Heart or Lung. Red on the edges suggests Heat in the Liver. Tooth marks on the edges indicate the tongue may be swollen — itself suggesting excess Dampness in the body. A pale tongue indicates a Yang deficiency — and a lack of Heat/(Summer) Heat. Finding a tongue both pale *and* marked by teeth suggests a combination of Dampness and Yang deficiencies.

---

[9]TCM doctors do recommend that patients avoid strong juices, coffee, and red wine prior to appointments, as these stain the tongue and mask the interpretive potential.

Regarding the coating of the tongue, doctors inspect the colour, thickness, dryness, texture, and distribution. A thin white coating is natural and healthy. A yellow coating, which many smokers possess, indicates Heat — especially external Heat: the darker/yellower the colour, the greater the degree of Heat. After a long-term illness, some patients lose all coating — in TCM, this is called 'mirror tongue', and it indicates 'Yin Exhaustion' which is a serious condition.

For the functioning of the tongue, the doctor will assess taste, movement, and speech. If the patient reports a lingering sweet taste, this could be a sign of excess Dampness or a weakness of the Spleen. A bitter taste could relate to a Liver problem, or to excess Heat. Abnormal or asymmetric movements could suggest a previous or pending stroke, or an excess of internal Wind.

2. Auscultation and Olfaction
Auscultation refers to a doctor's inspection of noises made by the patient's body — including the heart — typically by stethoscope. Olfaction refers to a doctor's inspection of a patient's smell. Between the two methods, doctors may develop a sense of the condition of the organs, as in TCM the sounds, noises, and odours all reflect upon the activity of those organs.

Speech: The coherence and fluency of speech are very much affected by the Shen and Qi. In TCM, the Heart controls the tongue and dominates the Shen. As such, incoherent speech indicates that the Heart-Shen is disturbed: excessively fast or slurred speech usually shows there is some Heat in the Heart, whereas unclear or illogical speech shows blockage of the Heart Qi, or Shen.

Voice: The Lung Qi and Zhong Qi[10] dominate the voice. If the voice is strong and loud, that means the patient is likely strong, or else suffers from syndromes of excess (of Heat, Cold, Damp, etc.). If the voice is weak, low, or strained the patient's Qi may be deficient. If the voice is heavy and deep, a Dampness may be blocking the Qi. Hoarseness indicates a blockage of both Heat and Phlegm, or Qi and Yin deficiency.

Coughing: In TCM, coughing is a symptom of the failure of the Lung to disperse Qi, permitting its flow. If Qi rises in the body, it results in coughing. Usually, this is caused by an invasion of external 'Evils', leading to a short period of coughing. A chronic or long-term cough indicates blockage, weakness, and/or lack of moisture in the Lung.

It is important to note that coughing can also be caused by the Heart, Liver, Spleen, and Kidney as well, because all these organs, if they are out of balance, can indirectly disturb the Lung Qi, resulting in the failure to descend and flow.

---

[10] See Glossary. Zhong Qi loosely translates to 'core' Qi — a combination of the Lung and Heart Qi, deep in the core of the body.

Coughing with phlegm suggests excess Dampness. If the phlegm is white in colour, it is 'Cold' phlegm, but if the phlegm is yellow in colour, it is 'Hot' phlegm. Coughing with little or no phlegm indicates a Yin deficiency.

Respiration: In TCM, breathing is controlled mainly by two organs: the Kidney and the Lung. Inhalation is controlled by the Kidney and exhalation by the lung. That is why shortness of breath, often seen in the elderly, is considered indicative of a weakness of the Kidney.

Rapid breathing is associated with Heat blockage, phlegm blockage, or with both — localised in the Lung. Wheezing is traditionally thought of as a Kidney weakness or Phlegm blockage, often caused by an incursion of Cold.

Belching: Belching indicates a weakness of the Spleen and Stomach. An improper diet can cause fermentation and gas production in the Stomach. In TCM, the Liver also plays an important role in digestion. If the Liver is overly restraining the Spleen and Stomach,[11] indigestion will occur, and the patient will belch. This can be

---

[11] As addressed in Chapter 2, in the Five Elements scheme, Liver is a Wood element, while the Spleen and Stomach are Earth elements: as Wood restrains Earth, so the Liver controls the digestion of the Stomach.

accompanied by acid reflux, and in many cases with pain, or a sensation of *fullness*.

Odours: Excessively offensive odours from the skin, mouth, nose, and body indicate stagnation of some kind: the organs' function of transportation and transformation of Qi has failed, leading to stagnation of either Qi, Blood, Body Waters, or food in the stomach.

The mal odour of stool or faeces is entirely normal. However, if this becomes too strong, especially together with other changes such as constipation or diarrhoea, it could mean that the Spleen and Stomach are out of tune: possibly due to indigestion or infection.

If the odour of urine is too strong, and there is difficulty in urinating, or an attendant burning sensation, this suggests there is a combined stagnation of Dampness and Heat. This usually corresponds to a urinary tract infection (UTI) in Western medicine.[12]

In infants especially, olfaction is an important diagnostic technique because of their limited ability to

---

[12]While on the subject of urine, there is an interesting TCM method for diagnosing high blood sugar problems and diabetes, which are referred to as 'Xiao Ke', or sugary urine diseases. Ancient TCM doctors would collect a sample of a patient's urine, put a few drops on the ground and place several ants near the urine. If the ants went to eat or drink the urine, this meant there was excessive sugar present: if the ants avoided the urine, it denoted a lack.

communicate. We therefore will often take care to check their faeces and urine.

3. Interrogation

Like the 'medical histories' taken in Western medicine, 'Interrogation' involves a set of exploratory discussions with the aim of discovering the nature and severity of a patient's complaint(s). At this stage, a doctor is also concerned with a patient's past medical conditions, their family's medical background, and the kinds of treatments and medications that have been or are being used.

Unlike Western 'medical histories', TCM Interrogation also seeks to reveal patient preferences: do they prefer hot or cold food, for example. Warm or cool environments? And so on. Such preferences can provide clues about the patient's conditions, be they Hot or Cold, Dry or Damp, etc.

Of course, such temperature preferences do not necessarily denote signs of fever, or low blood pressure, but simply what the patient is or is not comfortable with. Interrogation can involve a whole range of questions, and each line of questioning can be phrased in a host of different ways in order to cater to a patient's nature.[13]

---

[13] As in Western medicine, a strong interrogation is built upon a state of rapport/trust between doctor and patient. Not only must the patient feel at ease, such that they are willing to volunteer information but the conversation must also have the *space/room*

That said, most TCM experts identify the following ten core avenues that should be covered in a good TCM Interrogation, namely, whether the patient 'currently' has any of the following symptoms[14]:

- Feeling hot or cold;
- Sweating often, or too little;
- Experiencing head, chest, stomach, and generalised pains;
- Having difficulty urinating, or with bowel movements;
- Experiencing ear, eyes, nose, or throat symptoms;
- Coughing excessively;
- Excessively thirsty;
- Eating and drinking too little, too much, and of what;
- Experiencing symptoms related to the patient's medical history, or their familial medical history;

---

to expand into details that might seemingly — on first inspection — be irrelevant. For example, a good rapport might induce a patient to share with their doctor — once an appointment has concluded — that they have recently watched a certain television show they would recommend. A small detail like this might lead to a follow-up question — 'are you spending a lot of time watching television recently?' — which might in turn help to elicit highly relevant information, i.e., 'yes, more than usual — and I have been sleeping less as a result'. A good rapport provides space to better know all aspects of the patient: and knowing the patient is the foundation of diagnosis.

[14]In the present days and weeks — not necessarily in the present moment.

- Experiencing symptoms related to their menstrual cycle, pregnancy, or related condition(s).

Nowadays, a TCM doctor would want to move beyond these ten questions to cover further relevant subjects: but they still comprise the core basis of an Interrogation.

Contemporary extensions may then explore something like a patient's blood test results, scan results, or Western medical diagnosis. Western medical test results can, in fact, contribute good references or clues towards a patient's ultimate diagnosis in TCM: high cholesterol or high blood sugar level results, for example, can lead to a TCM diagnosis of Dampness and Kidney deficiency. In this way, we might begin to see the potential power of the Interrogation: sorting through the many possible clues to settle upon the strongest conclusion available.

4. Palpation and Pulse-Taking

As in a Western doctor's practice, TCM doctors also perform general palpation: the method of feeling with the hands during a physical examination. TCM doctors check, for example, for skin changes, for lumps and swelling, or for any signs of pain or tenderness. If a problem is superficial (for instance, a movable subdermal lump), then that usually indicates a milder degree of 'Qi' complaint. If the problem is deeper, findings may be classified as 'Blood'-level complaints.

Pulse-taking in TCM, on the other hand, is very different from that of Western medicine. Taking the pulse to obtain information about the rate and rhythm of the heart is an extremely common procedure in Western medicine, but in TCM doctors glean a much richer array of information: including the quality of the Blood and the status of its flow. Like tongue inspection, this is a skill that all TCM students learn: mastering it, however, is a long and difficult journey that few practitioners will ever truly complete.

In total, there are 28 different pulse types recognised in the literature, and these may vary in the same patient depending on the location the pulse is taken or on the time of day. It is therefore important to take frequent readings from the same patient: but more so, it is vital that doctors interpret the results as one small part of a greater whole — comprising all the aforementioned diagnostic methods — considering the meaning of any contradictory information in light of the entire dataset.

TCM teaches a general rule to help with differentiation between contradictory information. If the patient in question is suffering from seasonal illness, then doctors tend to use the tongue as a major criterion; if they suffer from a long-term chronic illness then pulse-taking is given more weight.

Critics remain sceptical on whether a practitioner can discern between these different types of pulses, and the potential insight into the quality of blood that pulse-taking can provide. To this, I would argue that training *can* sensitise one to subtle differences — differences that can be extrapolated through direct clinical experience. I have sat in the same North London office for years, and can now make a sensible inference of the kind of vehicle that passes underneath me through the differing patterns of vibration, without having to go out to the street to look, or to dig a hole under my desk to check.[15]

Part Three: Pulse-Taking

While the process of pulse-taking may be difficult to master, the principals are widely accessible: and given its importance to TCM diagnosis, it behoves us to briefly review the elements of the practice.

Location: In TCM, we take the pulse at the wrists, though in special circumstances we might also take the pulse at the neck or ankle.

The pulse is taken at both the left and the right wrists. Three fingers — the index, middle, and ring fingers — are placed simultaneously at the wrist. The index finger is placed closest to the hand — this position is called 'Cun'. The middle finger is next, in a position called

---

[15] Sitting in my office, blind to the truth of bus or train: am I right to be as confident as I am? Perhaps I *am* sometimes wrong — confident and ignorant regardless. But the years of practice make this rare: and the risk is exactly why TCM doctors triangulate such datapoints within the larger diagnostic whole.

'Guan', while the ring finger is placed at the back, closest to the elbow, a position called 'Chi'. These three positions reflect the upper, middle, and lower organs of the body, respectively, reflecting upon the health and status of those organs (see Table 1).

Table 1. Pulse and organ correspondence.

	Left Wrist Pulses	Right Wrist Pulses
Cun (index finger)	Heart Small intestine	Lung Large intestine
Guan (middle finger)	Liver Gallbladder	Spleen Stomach
Chi (ring finger)	Kidney Yin Urinary bladder	Kidney Yang Urinary bladder

Length: The pulse is differentiated by 'length', that is, the degree to which it is palpable across finger positions. Presence in all three (Cun, Guan, and Chi), or beyond, corresponds to a 'long' pulse, while presence in just one or two corresponds to 'short' pulse. A long pulse indicates healthy Qi flow or Liver Yang hyperactivity, whereas a short pulse indicates contraction or deficiency of Qi and Liver Qi stagnation.

Timing: Tradition holds that the best time to take the pulse is in the morning. Immediately after waking, the body's Yin Qi and Yang Qi are still quite settled and have not yet been subject to the disturbances that naturally affect heart rate, blood pressure, and pulse.

Rate: A TCM doctor will normally spend 3 to 4 minutes studying each wrist. TCM pulse rate examinations were developed in ancient China before doctors had access to clocks and watches. Without such tools, doctors used their own breathing rate to count the pulse: if there were 4 to 5 beats between each breath, this was considered a normal rate; over 5, and the rate was too fast, and below 4, too slow.[16] A fast pulse is indicative of excessive Heat, while a slow pulse suggests excessive Cold.

Rhythm: TCM considers regularity a basic concept of a healthy life. We see this played out across the natural world in the regular cycles of plant and animal life, and the same rule applies to the pulse.

The following types of irregular pulse, or rhythm break, may indicate health issues:

1. Intermittent pulse: An irregular and intermittent pulse indicates a disturbance in Qi and Blood, the exhaustion of organs, or trauma.

2. Hurried pulse: A rapid, irregular, and intermittent pulse indicates an invasion of Heat in the Heart, or else

---

[16] This technique corresponds to a Western understanding of physiology. A healthy adult heart rate is approximately 60 to 90 beats per minute, while a healthy adult breathing rate is about 15 to 18 breaths per minute, giving a ratio of 4 to 5 beats per breath.

excessive Heat in the body that has led to stagnation of both Qi and Blood.

3. Knotted pulse: A slow, irregular, and intermittent pulse indicates an invasion of Cold in the Heart, Cold obstruction, the blockage of Qi at meridians, or a Heart Qi or Heart Yang deficiency.

Depth: During the pulse-taking procedure, a doctor will apply three different levels of pressure: light, medium, and heavy. The depth at which the pulse can be felt most strongly indicates the depth of an illness — should an illness be if present. The three states are as follows:

1. Floating pulse: Palpable at a superficial level; indicating an exterior syndrome or Qi deficiency.

2. Medium pulse: Palpable at a medium level, which indicates a healthy body.

3. Sinking pulse: Palpable at a deep level, indicating an interior syndrome.

For example, when 'Wind-Cold' or 'Wind-Heat' is present in superficial parts of the body, such as the throat or nose, a patient may complain of flu or cold symptoms — and the pulse is likely to be 'floating'. A doctor would then treat this by inducing sweating to expel the Wind-Cold or Wind-Heat.

However, if the pulse is 'sinking', then this suggests the condition is more severe, with the 'Wind-Cold' or

'Wind-Heat' having invaded deeper parts of the body, such as the lungs.

Force: The 'bouncing' force of the pulse can indicate the strength of the body's Qi and Blood. TCM therefore differentiates between a 'Strong' and a 'Weak' pulse.

Quality: Assessing the quality of the pulse involves examining its shape, fullness, thickness, and flexibility. The most common types of pulse are described as 'Slippery', 'Wiry', and 'Choppy'.

1. Slippery: Feels like a ball rolling under your fingers, because the Blood is thick or rich and full. Phlegm, Dampness, and food stagnation are often associated with this pulse. One's pulse is usually Slippery during pregnancy — it's considered a good sign by TCM doctors and may be a result of a larger volume of Blood.

2. Wiry: Feels like touching a thin wire — narrow, stringy, rebounding against pressure, like plucking the strings of a violin. A wiry pulse is associated with Liver problems and emotional stress. Patients with clinical depression commonly have this kind of pulse. Other associated problems include Qi stagnation, Gallbladder disorders, muscle pain, and menstrual problems.

3. Choppy: Has been described as feeling 'like shaving bamboo with a knife' (as per the ancient TCM manuals): sluggish, uneven, hesitant. This indicates a rough, uneven flow of Blood associated with Qi and Blood deficiency, stagnation of Qi and Blood, and Blood loss.

How Many Pulses are There in TCM?

There is no definitive number of pulses in TCM, as figures vary from text to text. Most describe 20 to 28 different types. Table 2 summarises the most common, some of which I have already described above.

Table 2. Pulse types in TCM.

Pulse Name	Description
Floating	Palpable on a superficial level. Indicates exterior syndrome or Qi deficiency.
Sinking	Palpable on a deep level. Indicates interior syndrome.
Slow	Fewer than 4 beats per respiration. Indicates Cold syndrome or Yang deficiency.
Rapid	More than 5 beats per respiration. Indicates Heat syndrome or Yin deficiency.
Weak	Empty, without strength. Indicates a deficiency syndrome.
Strong	Full and vibrant. Indicates a syndrome of excess.
Thin	Thread-like. Indicates Blood deficiency.
Big	Forceful. Indicates a syndrome of excess, Heat in the Stomach or Intestines.
Slippery	Fluid, like beads fast rolling on a plate. Indicates phlegm, dampness, food stagnation, and Heat. Can also be a healthy pulse.
Choppy	Sluggish, uneven, hesitant. Indicates Qi and Blood deficiency, or stagnation of both.
Wiry	Taut, stringy, rebounds against pressure. Indicates Liver and Gallbladder disorder, Qi stagnation, and muscle pain.
Tight	Tense; bounces from side to side like a taut rope. Indicates Cold syndrome or pain.

Table 2. (*Continued*)

Pulse Name	Description
Short	Short duration. Indicates contraction of Qi (Liver Qi stagnation) or deficient Qi.
Long	Perceptible beyond three finger positions. Indicates Liver Yang hyperactivity.
Knotted	Slow pulse pausing at irregular intervals — indicating Cold obstruction, Qi blockage at the meridians, or Heart Qi deficiency.
Hurried	Rapid pulse with irregular intermittence. Indicates excessive Heat with stagnation of Qi and Blood.
Intermittent	Slow pulse pausing at regular intervals. Indicating a declining Heart Qi and Blood, exhaustion of organs, and trauma.
Relaxed and Soft	Diminished tension. Indicating weakness of Qi and obstruction through Damp.
Flooding	Beating, like dashing waves, forcefully rising and gradually falling. Indicates a syndrome of excess.
Minute	Thready, soft, scarcely perceptible, on the edge of disappearing. Indicates extreme deficiency.
Frail	Soft, weak, thin. Indicates serious deficiency of Qi and Blood.
Soggy	Thin, empty, floating. Indicates deficiency of Blood or Jing; associated with Dampness syndrome.
Leather	Wiry, floating, and empty. Indicates deficiency of Blood and/or Jing.
Hidden	An extreme form of a deep pulse. Felt at the bone. Indicates Cold syndrome, syncope, or severe pain.

Part Four: Analysis and Decision-Making

When a patient visits a TCM doctor, they will invariably be told they have some manner of 'syndrome'. The TCM doctor may tell a patient with eczema, like J, for example, that they have a 'Heat syndrome' or a 'Damp-Heat syndrome'. The patient may further be told they have a 'deficiency syndrome' of an organ like the Kidney. This kind of terminology is very different from the language of the Western medical clinic.

What is a syndrome in TCM? We use the word syndrome to mean a collection of symptoms and signs, organised by a cause or family of causes. Making a diagnosis in TCM is the consistent process of differentiation between syndromes.

Critics argue that the syndrome represents a vague, imprecise, and out-of-date concept. Diagnostic precision can be a positive thing, of course, but from the TCM perspective, that precision can often sacrifice the holistic understanding of a bigger picture. To the TCM doctor, J's eczema was not only an infection of the skin, a breast cancer not just a tumour in tissue: to believe otherwise risks blinding oneself to a network of connective meanings, and to the unity of the body's many systems. In that discourse between scientific precision on the one hand and systemic totality on the other, a TCM doctor opts for the latter.

Differentiating between different syndromes means analysing and categorising all the information one has gathered about the patient. Reflecting upon the many signs, symptoms, and histories — one may begin to determine the possible cause, nature, and severity of a sickness: its internal relations, potential consequences, and the state of conflict between 'Vital' and 'Evil' Qi. Only by studious differentiation between syndromes can a TCM doctor fix an effective treatment that accords to the condition of the disease.

Syndromes are structured, differentiated, and classified in several different ways by the great authors of the tradition. Key among these is the 'Eight Principal Syndromes' through which all conditions can be classified. Other methods of classification include the following:

- The organ syndromes;
- Changes to Qi, Blood, and Body Waters[17];
- The 'Four Levels', or Wei, Qi, Ying, and Xue (Blood);
- The 'Six Divisions': Tai Yang Syndrome, Shao Yang Syndrome, Yang Ming Syndrome, Tai Yin Syndrome, Shao Yin Syndrome, and Jue Yin Syndrome.[18]

We will soon address these classifications in greater detail.

---

[17]These apply more specifically to internal disorders.
[18]These apply more specifically to feverish disorders.

The Eight Principal Syndromes

The Eight Principal Syndromes refer to Yin and Yang, Exterior and Interior, Cold and Heat, and degrees of deficiency and excess. It is important to note that:

- Interior, Cold, and Deficiency syndrome are generally related to Yin;
- Exterior, Heat, and Excess syndromes generally relate to Yang.

Therefore, Yin and Yang serve as representative 'headings' of the other syndromes.

Exterior and Interior Syndromes

In simple terms, 'Exterior' and 'Interior' refer to the location of a pathology — superficial on the one hand, deep on the other. However, the theory becomes more complex as we consider that External and Internal are defined *relative to one another*. From one perspective, the skin may be considered Exterior while other organs, Interior, while in another case the Zang (hollow) organs may be considered Exterior, while the Fu (solid) organs Interior. In other words, Exterior and Interior exist as two terminals of a continuum. In general, however, we tend to draw the line between the two at the level of the Zang organs, thereby classifying the Zang organs, Fu organs, Blood, and bone marrow as Interior, while the skin, muscles, and meridians are classified as Exterior.

The depth of a disease reflects a measure of its severity — for example, as a disease invades into deeper parts of the body, the farther it progresses, the greater the severity. Equally, the movement of a disease from deep to superficial parts suggests an improvement in a patient's condition.

Accurate differentiation between Exterior and Interior syndromes helps not only when establishing the correct treatment but also in understanding the development and progress of that disease.

Exterior syndrome is characterised by a sudden onset, superficial location, mild symptoms, and a short course. It is usually seen in the initial stages when the 'Six Evils' — Wind, Cold, Summer-Heat, Dampness, Dryness, and Heat — invade the body and obstruct the normal dispersion of defensive (or Wei) Qi. Resistance by Vital (or Zhen) Qi leads to some of the clinical manifestations of Exterior syndrome including fever, aversion to cold, headache, general body aches, a runny nose, sore throat, cough, thin and white tongue coating, and a floating pulse.

Interior syndrome is characterised by complex causation, deep location, varied symptoms, and a more severe and prolonged course. It covers a wide range of diseases, including those where the 'Six Evils' have been transmitted from the Exterior to the Zang and Fu organs; it is associated with the internal causes of disease, such as the 'Seven Emotions', inappropriate diets and levels of work, and direct damage to the Zang and Fu organs. The syndrome usually co-occurs with other syndromes — Cold or Heat, Deficiency or Excess. Common symptoms include high fever, thirst, abdominal pain, constipation, diarrhoea, vomiting, scanty dark urine, irritability, a thick tongue coating, a deep pulse, and even coma.

For infectious diseases, the depth of infection is divided more specifically than just Interior and Exterior. The classification consists of four levels. The first level is called 'Wei' which in Chinese means 'defence' and often stands at the early stage of an infection, such as early symptoms of the common cold or flu, before the virus has gotten into the lungs. The second level is 'Qi' — in the example of the flu, this would arise when the virus is just starting to express itself in the lungs. The third level is 'Ying' — the infectious agent hasn't reached the level of the Blood yet, but will start to show some related symptoms, such as coughing up thick phlegm, or purple skin rashes. The fourth level is 'Xue', or 'Blood' — this represents late stages of an infection and is characterised by changes to the 'Shen' or spirit, such as delirium or coma. This is because Blood directly connects to the Heart, which houses the Shen.

Cold and Heat Syndromes

Zhang Jing-Yue, a famous TCM doctor of the Tang Dynasty, explained that 'Cold and Heat syndromes are manifestations of Yin–Yang changes'.

'Cold syndrome' is often caused by a deficiency of Yang and/or an excess of Yin in the body, or by an impairment of Yang due to prolonged illness. It can also be caused by an invasion of pathogenic Cold: one of the Six Evils. Exterior Cold Syndrome is characterised by an aversion to cold, mild fever without sweat, headache and body ache, thin white coating of the tongue, and a floating and tense pulse, whereas Interior Cold Syndrome is characterised by cold intolerance, cold limbs, pale complexion, loss of taste, profuse salivation, copious clear urine, loose stool, a pale tongue with white moist coating, and a deep, slow pulse.

'Heat syndrome' indicates functional hyperactivity of the body, arising from an invasion of pathogenic Heat, Fire transformation from a disorder of the emotions, or from an improper diet. The weakness of Qi and Yin can lead to internal Heat too. Exhaustion of Yin and Essence (Jing) will also cause Yang and, consequently, Heat to rise. Heat can also occur after the initial invasion of external Cold, where the Cold, once inside the body, transforms into Heat. Like Cold syndrome, Heat syndrome is also divided according to location into Exterior and Interior syndromes. Furthermore, however, Heat can be differentiated according to the strength of the Qi and Blood, and according to Deficiency and Excess, as explained at the end of this chapter.

Heat syndromes are characterised by a red face, red tongue, aversion to heat and a rapid pulse. Exterior Heat is also marked by fever, thirst, a yellow coating on the tongue, dark urine, yellow phlegm, skin rashes, mucus, or even bleeding. Interior Heat is marked by insomnia, restlessness, dry skin, dry mouth, and constipation.

Cold and Heat syndromes can present additional complexity. Symptoms that appear as manifestations of Heat can occur in the Cold syndrome, and we call these 'pseudo-Heat' symptoms. Meanwhile, the opposite is true for 'pseudo-Cold' symptoms. When differentiating between Cold and Heat syndromes, we should therefore analyse all the symptoms and signs present, rather than jump to conclusions based on isolated symptoms.

Deficiency and Excess Syndromes

As discussed previously, illness arises due to an imbalance of the body's Vital Qi (Zhen Qi) and Evil Qi. If there is weakness in the Vital Qi, illness will arise — if this is mild or temporary, the illness will be short-term, but if the weakness is more severe, we call this a 'Deficiency' syndrome.

In contrast, an 'Excess' syndrome arises mainly due to strong Evil Qi. Sometimes, there is a combination of a weak Vital Qi and strong Evil Qi, but we tend to label the syndrome as Deficiency or Excess depending on what the dominant factor is.

The weakness of Vital Qi in Deficiency syndromes can be caused by inherited weakness, an improper lifestyle and diet, or inappropriate treatment. It can be divided into Exterior or Interior, Qi or Blood, Yin, or Yang and by the organ affected.

Symptoms of Deficiency syndrome vary depending on where and what is deficient. For example, a Heart deficiency will manifest with palpitations, Spleen deficiency with poor digestion and loose stool, *or* Kidney deficiency with frequent urination and lower back pain.

Certain symptoms are common across Deficiency syndromes: tiredness, poor appetite, shallow breathing, low voice, weak muscles, and a pale complexion. The pulse in some or all locations is weak, and the tongue is pale and lacks coating.

In Excess syndromes, Evil Qi can include external factors such as the Six Evils, or internal factors, such as the Seven Emotions — or internal Phlegm, Dampness, or stagnated Blood. Excess syndrome can be further divided into Exterior or Interior, Hot or Cold, or according to its location in a specific organ — the symptoms will vary accordingly.

Excess syndrome mainly occurs in Fu (hollow) organs like the Stomach, Intestines, and Bladder, and rarely in Zang (solid) organs like the Heart, Spleen, and Kidney, because they are protected by their location in the interior of the body. However, if Zang organs are affected by strong Evil Qi, then TCM would consider this a serious condition. Despite variability in symptoms, the most common symptom in Excess syndromes is pain: this tends to be strong, fixed in location and tender to the touch. The pulse of the patient will be strong, and the tongue will normally have a thick coating.

Yin and Yang Syndromes

The most fundamental differentiation of illness is into Yin and Yang syndromes. Yang syndromes tend to combine Exterior, Heat, and Excess syndromes. Signs and symptoms therefore include fever, red complexion, restlessness, a high-pitched voice, hoarse breath, dry mouth, thirst, dark yellow urine, retention of dry faeces, a red tongue with a thick yellow coating, and a fast, strong pulse.

In opposition to this is the Yin syndrome, which tends to combine Interior, Cold, and Deficiency syndromes, thus manifesting with cold limbs, a pale complexion, dispiritedness, fatigue, a low-pitched voice, shortness of breath, a bland taste in the mouth, lack of thirst, clear and profuse urine, loose stool, pale and tender tongue with white coating, and a slow, weak pulse.

However, in clinical practice, Yin and Yang syndromes do not always map on to Exterior, Interior, Heat, Cold, Excess, or Deficiency syndromes with unwavering consistency. This is because Yin and Yang are defined relative to one another, and — crucially — because in TCM these forces also shift and transform *into* the other: making boundaries fluid and ill defined.

The skilled TCM doctor therefore needs to identify the dominant presence of either Yin or Yang from the variety of signs and symptoms present: once achieved, the doctor can judge the status of the illness, and the prognosis at large.

Qi, Blood, and Body Water Syndromes

Another important method of classification involves the study of pathological change in Qi, Blood, and Body Waters. This classification scheme identifies three families of illness: issue of quantity; issue of movement; and issue of quality.

Issues of Quantity

Deficiency in Qi, Blood, and/or Body Water usually arises due to a problem in quality, but can also arise in physical loss or reduced production.

The three variants are as follows:

- *Qi deficiency*: This can apply to either general Qi or to the Qi of individual organs, resulting in varied symptoms. Common symptoms include tiredness, feeling cold, a pale complexion, a pale — or swollen and wet — tongue, and a weak, slow pulse.
- *Blood deficiency*: Applying either to general 'Blood', or to the Blood of individual organs: most commonly the Heart, Liver, and Spleen. Symptoms include a pale or sallow complexion, tiredness,

palpitations, a pale, dry tongue, and a weak but fast pulse.

- *Body Water deficiency*: This applies only generally, rather than to specific organs. However, body fluid quantity issues often occur together with Blood deficiency, and/or Yin deficiency, because Body Water is associated with Yin. The common symptoms are dryness of skin, mouth, and throat, thirst and weight loss, a dry tongue, and weak, thin, and fast pulse.

Issues of Movement

Qi, Blood, and Body Water can also malfunction because of difficulties in flow. Normal circulation has a smooth flow and follows certain directions and speeds, though this can be disrupted in several ways:

- *Qi stagnation*: When the flow of Qi is too slow or uneven, this can result in a partial or complete blockage, or in other words, 'stagnation'. This is a frequent and potent cause of pain. We therefore treat pain by trying to unblock the stagnation through acupuncture, massage, or herbal medicines — this is arguably very different from Western medicine, where pain treatment is designed to block nerve transmissions. Pain secondary to Qi stagnation characteristically moves around — or else is not fixed in one place — and is not tender to palpation. The tongue may appear normal or dull and the pulse is usually wiry.
- *Blood stagnation*: Similar to Qi stagnation, Blood stagnation arises due to the slow or uneven flow of

Blood but can be also caused by a dominant Qi stagnation: resulting in pain. As Blood is at a deeper level than Qi, stagnation of Blood is generally more serious than the stagnation of Qi, and it leads to a more severe pain — sharp in nature, fixed in location, and tender to touch, potentially with palpable lumps. Patients with Blood stagnation will normally have a longer history of illness than the Qi stagnation alone. In women, it can also lead to dark menstrual bleeding, with the potential for blood clots. The tongue is usually dark or covered with purple patches, and the pulse is wiry.

- *Body Water retention*: When Body Water moves too slowly, or there is a blockage, this results in water retention and swelling. Those suffering from Body Water retention tend to have a wet or swollen tongue with a thick coating and a deep pulse. In TCM, the flow of Body Water is controlled by the Lung, Spleen, and Kidney. Disturbed Water retention means a problem with those organs, one of them or all three. The related symptoms and signs of those organs provide the clues.

- *Qi sinking*: When Qi fails to move upwards and rise to upper parts of the body, it descends or sinks. This is often resultant from deficiency in the quality of Qi, and most commonly affects the Spleen Qi. Sinking Qi is characterised by the prolapse of organs, such as the stomach, rectum, and/or uterus. Patients also feel tired and dizzy and may experience chronic diarrhoea. A pale tongue and weak pulses are common.

- *Qi ascending*: When Qi fails to move downwards, it moves upwards or 'ascends'. This often refers specifically to the Liver, Lung, or Stomach Qi, and leads to characteristic 'ascending' symptoms: coughing in ascending Lung Qi, hiccupping, belching in ascending Stomach Qi, and headaches and tinnitus in ascending Liver Qi. In serious cases of ascending Liver Qi, the patients may feel dizzy, faint, vomit blood, or even lapse into a coma.

Issues of Quality

- *Hot Blood*: As described previously, Hot and Cold syndromes can also apply specifically to the Blood. 'Hot Blood' results in a flushed face, skin rashes, dry skin, a rapid pulse, a red tongue, nose bleeds, bleeding gums, and, for women, heavy menstrual bleeding. If there is bleeding, the blood is usually fresh, red, and thin (unlike the darker, clotted blood in Blood stagnation and 'Cold Blood'). This can arise due to either external or internal Heat.
- *Cold Blood*: When Cold attacks Blood, it causes Blood stagnation, thus resulting in the previously mentioned symptoms, including pain and dark, clotted menstrual bleeding. Many people, especially women, suffer from Cold Blood syndrome in winter. In layman's terms, one could call it 'bad circulation': they might feel cold, especially in their hands and feet. Other signs include period pains and even Raynaud's syndrome — where fingers and toes change colour because of poor blood supply. However,

unlike other causes of Blood stagnation, these symptoms will improve if the patient is able to get warm. The tongue is usually pale and the pulse slow. Cold Blood syndrome can be caused by exterior Cold and/or an internal Yang deficiency.

* *Internal dampness and phlegm*: When Body Waters are thick and sticky, they will not flow smoothly, resulting in an Internal Dampness syndrome. Symptoms include swelling and puffiness, oedema, weight gain, loose stool, tiredness, and a heavy feeling in the head.

The tongue is swollen and pale with a thick coating, while the pulse is slippery. They are both caused by a bad quality of Body Waters. The terms of Internal Dampness and Phlegm can be interchangeable, the symptoms and signs of which can be very similar — sometimes difficult to distinguish. Phlegm is a more extreme but localised manifestation of Internal Dampness. In TCM, Phlegm can be both visible and invisible — in the Lungs, visible mucus causes coughing or wheezing, but invisible Phlegm can also seep into the meridians, causing numbness or paralysis, or leading to lumps or tumours.

Organ Syndromes

The Heart, Lung, Spleen, Liver, and Kidney are the five key organs of the body, and together make up the innermost core. They work together as a whole, but also dominate specific functions of the body. All illnesses will be linked to each of these five organs, though to differing proportions and degrees.

Heart Syndrome

The most common Heart syndromes are Heart Qi deficiencies and Heart Blood deficiencies. The symptoms include a lack of energy, shallow breathing, palpitations, chest pain, insomnia, spontaneous sweating, and a weak pulse. The tongue is usually pale or red, without a coating.

Lung Syndrome

The most common Lung syndromes are a Lung Qi deficiency, Wind-Cold in the Lung, and Heat and/or Phlegm blocking the Lung. The symptoms can include coughing, wheezing, a blocked nose, increased mucus and phlegm, difficulty in breathing, losing one's voice, constipation, and sometimes fluid in the lungs. The pulse can be floating, fast, or weak. The tongue is pale or red, with a white or yellow coating, depending on the precise nature of the problem.

Spleen Syndrome

The most common Spleen syndromes are Spleen Qi deficiencies, Spleen Yang deficiencies, and the sinking of Spleen Qi. The symptoms usually include tiredness, poor appetite, abdominal distension, stomach pain, loose stool or diarrhoea, prolapse of stomach, rectum, or uterus, dizziness, low voice, excessive vaginal discharge, fluid build-up, increased amounts of mucus, and a weak, slow, or slippery pulse. The tongue is pale and swollen, marked with teeth marks; the coating is thick and white.

Liver Syndrome

The most common Liver syndromes are Liver Qi and/ or Blood stagnation, and Liver Blood or Liver Yin deficiency. The symptoms can include low mood, migratory pain in the chest, breast tenderness or lumps, irregular menstruation, menstrual pain, dizziness, dry eyes, poor vision, fever, a lack of energy, numbness, and weak nails and hair. The pulse can be wiry or weak. The tongue is usually pale or red, with a lack of coating.

Kidney Syndrome

The most common Kidney syndromes are Kidney Qi or Yang deficiency, and Kidney Yin deficiency. Symptoms include a long-term lack of energy, shallow breathing, back and knee pain, dizziness, tinnitus, amnesia, night sweats, and low sexual energy with a weak and thin pulse. The tongue is pale and swollen, or red and dry, characterised by cracks and peeling, without much coating.

Chapter 6

Treatment of Illness in TCM

Part One: Branches and Roots

TCM does not recognise illness — even pathogenic illness — as a discrete phenomenon. Rather, it is understood as the wave of consequences that emanate from a posture of imbalance. Treatment, therefore, is the practice and process of restoring that balance; rather than simply addressing that wave, or the damage done in its wake, treatments in TCM seek to settle it at the source.[1]

TCM is not alone here, and there are parallels in certain Western treatment plans. Diabetes therapy, for example, involves a habitual and active balance of blood sugar levels through the daily administration of insulin. Indeed, Western doctors would treat chronic hormone syndromes — such as those brought on by excessive or inadequate presence of hormones — through the

---

[1] This relates back to the concept of 'Root Treatment'. See Glossary for more information.

rebalancing of hormone levels by additive daily prescription.

However, it should be acknowledged that Western medical practice usually considers an illness *as such*. That is to say, its diagnosis and subsequent treatment considers the illness as a discrete form, rather than a resultant expression of a form abstracted. Focusing on identifying and solving a perceived 'problem' — an infection or tumour, for example — the root causes of that problem are not contained within the boundaries of the exercise.[2]

In TCM, symptoms and problems are considered the superficial manifestations of an illness: what we call the 'Biao' — which can be translated as 'branches' or 'leaves'. The tradition holds that a focus on only treating the Biao thereby ignores the internal conditions that predisposed the body to that infection or tumour in the first place; we call this the 'Ben' (or the 'roots').

When removing weeds, a master gardener will pull not only the leaves but also the roots to ensure what is

---

[2] This is not to claim that Western medicine never considers cause. Whole fields of epidemiology exist that tackle the causes of certain diseases, while some medical care — especially care in which resources are not a limiting factor — may address the question of cause once a treatment plan has been established (think dietary referrals). Nevertheless, it *can* be said that Western medicine's problem-oriented method does not contain the inquiry into *cause* as a definitive part of that method.

unwanted will not regrow. By treating the Ben, a doctor not only addresses the Biao but denies the conditions that create it.

In the Tradition, the root (or Ben) of an illness is the state of imbalance in the body's Qi, Yin, and Yang. Often, this will seem far removed from the Biao. Consider for example a patient of mine who once suffered from tinnitus. When I first saw him, he reported frequent hot flushes at night, and passing large amounts of urine; his tongue was red and cracked. The 'Ben' in this case was a Kidney Yin deficiency. In other words, the body's fluids — here acting as a cooling system — were not flowing properly, and the excess Heat was drying out his organs and nerves, leading to the tinnitus. I advised him to avoid certain foods, coffee, and alcohol, provided several acupuncture sessions, and prescribed cooling herbs to nourish his Kidneys. A devoted student of the Western school might raise an eyebrow at my suggestion that the underlying root of an ear problem was in the Kidneys: but in TCM, where the body is always viewed as an interconnected whole, this is par for the course.

After a few weeks, the night sweats stopped, and the patient's tinnitus greatly improved. By diagnosing and tackling the Ben, my aim was to shift the internal environment such that the body was able to heal itself. In TCM, great emphasis is placed on this incredible ability to heal and adapt. Indeed, in the Tradition, this is the only way to truly 'cure' an illness: even the best doctors will only ever play a guiding role — fine-tuning and rebalancing to promote and secure.

Prior to visiting me, the patient's tinnitus was diagnosed as a localised ear disorder and treated with suction and antibiotics by a Western doctor. The tinnitus only worsened; if a gardener *only* removes stalks and branches, these weeds can regrow stronger.

I often see patients who have experienced recurrent infections and have received multiple courses of antibiotics. While counterintuitive to the Western mind, from a TCM perspective, it *can* be the repeated use of these antibiotics that increases a body's susceptibility to future infections. By weakening various organs through their side effects, providing artificial supports that displace existing defensive forces, and offsetting the body's internal balance, a demonstrably effective chemical, like antibiotics, can nevertheless *increase* our vulnerability over time.[3]

There will be times when the Biao is the immediate priority: a patient with dangerously low or high blood pressure will need treatment as an emergency. When a patient has a fast-growing cancer, timely removal is often advised to prevent serious complications. Sooner or later, however, a TCM doctor will always need to

---

[3] Do not take this to mean that a TCM practitioner denies the efficacy of penicillin. The difference here relates less to understanding than it does method, perspective, and scale.

turn to the Ben in order to promote healing and prevent recurrence.[4]

As outlined in Chapter 1, the methods of treatment within TCM are varied. A course of treatment will usually also involve one or more of the following:

• Herbal medicines
• Acupuncture
• Cupping
• Dietary and lifestyle instruction
• Moxibustion
• Qi Gong
• Tai Chi
• Massage

Acupuncture

I am often asked how acupuncture works. TCM theory posits that the insertion of very fine needles into certain points along the meridians can stimulate the body's healing response, helping to stimulate the flow of Qi, in turn restoring the conditions of balance. As the Qi of each organ travels to and acts within all parts of the body, an acupuncturist may fruitfully insert needles into

---

[4]I suspect that Western medicine is gradually coming around to this too — oncologists, for instance, increasingly recognise the role of a weak immune system in the development of cancer — appreciating the predisposing conditions which allow cancer to arise.

an area that is not obviously related to the location of the symptoms.

Qi Gong and Tai Chi

Qi Gong and Tai Chi are exercise therapies that combine static postures and rhythmic movements with meditation and breathing. They activate the body's internal systems to promote the circulation of Qi, Blood, and Body Water. This leads to an increased feeling of vitality in healthy people and promotes healing in the sick.

Dietary and Lifestyle Instruction

A course of treatment for all conditions will, to a greater or lesser extent, involve lifestyle changes. This can include changes to diet, exercise, sleep, or other behaviours and attitudes. The treatment process is one of partnership, and requires the patient to apply themselves. Here, we return to the TCM beliefs that emphasise the role of self-healing.

A 'good' diet is a relative thing. Each food has a particular property — Hot,[5] Warm, Cool, Cold, etc. These properties partly derive from the origins of the food in question — with origins near water associated with cold or cool properties, near mountains with warm or

---

[5] *Not* 'hot' in terms of spice!

hot.[6] Cooking methods can change or modify the properties of food: frying brings heat, whereas steaming brings cooling and damp. The properties of food act on specific organs and their functions. Hot and warm food usually speeds up the movements of Qi, or the functions of organs, whereas cold and cool foods do the opposite. Equally, our five essential tastes reflect the Five Elements theory, wherein naturally sweet foods tend to benefit the Spleen, bitter foods the Heart, sour foods the Liver, pungent foods the Lung, and salty foods the Kidney. Food also has an energising action that can strengthen specific organs or meridians, altering the balances of their Qi and Blood.

By understanding the action, taste, and property of foods, a practitioner may recommend the inclusion or exclusion of specific foods under specific conditions: carefully illustrating a 'good' diet as that which leads most directly back to a holistic balance.

Part Two: Herbal Medicines

Herbal medicine is a highly important, if complex part of TCM treatment. The Tradition applies over 8000 herbs, with many hundreds of thousands of classical combinations (or *formulae*) in the TCM Pharmacopoeia. The plants in question all have an

---

[6]I explore the nature of different foods at greater length in Chapter 7.

effect on the body's Qi. Some herbs have the property of Heat, others Cold, some are Dry, and others Damp. Herbal formulae can generally be categorised according to the Eight Principal theory to describe the ways through which they enhance or regulate Qi, inducing sweating, vomiting, defecation, warming, clearing, tonifying, harmonising, and 'reducing'.

Sweating

Some herbs or herbal formulae induce sweating by stimulating Lung Qi and Wei Qi (Defensive Qi). They aim to open the pores, expelling pathogenic influences or 'Evils' through sweat. When Cold invades the body through the skin, this can close the pores, so that the Evil is unable to be expelled so moves deeper into the body, such as into the Lungs. Therefore, in the early stages of a Wind-Cold or Cold-Damp syndrome, where a patient has the early symptoms of a cold or a flu, it is particularly important to induce sweating. I often advise patients at this stage to drink plenty of hot water and fresh ginger tea, as ginger is a warming herb that induces sweating. Hot showers, saunas, and even a little spiciness in food are beneficial here.

The sweating treatment method must be gentle: overdoing it can cause harm, weakening the body's Qi and Yin, which can lead to a delay in healing or a worsening of the sickness. We therefore advise that the degree of sweat should create a slight dampness at the skin — profuse and heavy sweating should be avoided.

Vomiting

When certain poisons or toxic foods have been consumed, or when digestion functions poorly and food remains stagnant or fermenting in the stomach, patients may complain of bloating, pain, belching, bad breath, or constipation. To eliminate such toxic or stagnant stomach contents, we can use herbal formulae to induce vomiting. However, this is an uncommon method of treatment because of how unpleasant an experience it is, and because it can injure the Stomach and throat Qis. Therefore, it should only be used for treating acute disorders in relatively robust patients.

Defecation or 'Draining Downwards'

Defecation can be induced to cleanse the bowels and expel substantive pathogenic Evils through the rectum. In TCM, regular bowel movements are important to the maintenance of health and improper bowel movements can be a major cause of imbalance in the body. TCM holds that slow bowel movements lead to stagnation and fermentation, which can become poisonous to the body. Inducing defecation through certain herbal formulae, through a process we also call 'Draining Downwards', helps to purge this stagnant food, and can also purge Evils such as Heat out of the body. Unlike some modern methods, such as colonic irrigation, this method is internal, natural, and cleanses the whole digestive system — not just the large intestines.

As with vomiting, doctors must also be careful when inducing defecation so as to avoid diarrhoea and the weakening of the Spleen.

Warming

For internal Cold syndrome caused by Qi and Yang deficiency, warming herbs can be used to unblock channels and dispel Cold from the organs, thereby restoring the function of Yang Qi and preventing further complications, such as Blood stagnation.

Clearing

Internal Heat syndrome often progresses in severity, transforming into Fire if it is left unaddressed, damaging Body Waters, Yin, and even Qi. Clearing Heat is therefore essential. Herbs which do this often promote urination to reach this end. As Heat often damages Yin, we usually also recommend simultaneous use of herbs that nourish Yin.

Tonifying

Using tonifying herbs to enrich, nurture, or replenish those aspects of the body that are weak or deficient is the most common application of herbs.

In the clinic, I use herbs with precision and purpose to target root deficiencies. Importantly, I also advise not using supplemental vitamins, minerals, and nourishing treatments alongside a treatment plan. As we have explored, TCM maintains that once the root deficiency is resolved, other deficiencies will naturally self-heal; under these conditions, unintended supplements will only serve to confuse and slow the return path to balance. Overusing or hurrying treatments can also cause long-term damage to the Spleen and Liver, further weakening the body.

Deficiencies of the body can be divided into those of Qi, Blood, Yin, and Yang, and these can affect various organs. Different herbal formulae target different deficiencies, though most are supplemented with a Spleen tonic, as the Spleen is the key organ dominating digestion, absorption, and dissemination. As these tonics are usually sweet and Damp in nature, this itself must be rebalanced by the use of other herbs.

Harmonising

In TCM, 'harmonising' means to regulate and balance. While all TCM treatments aim to restore balance, harmonising treatments in particular focus on the balance of Qi and Blood, especially the Liver Qi and Spleen Qi, as these have major control over the body's Qi and Blood. Attaining harmony between the Liver and Spleen is an essential precondition to healing many illnesses.

Reducing

If the stagnation of food, Phlegm, Qi, or Blood is new or acute, then purging techniques can be usefully applied (i.e., vomiting; defecation). However, for a more lasting or solid stagnation, we apply the 'reducing' method to gradually clear the excessive accumulation. This can be particularly effective in chronic or resident diseases, such as abscesses or tumours, where application of specific 'reducing' herbs serves to eliminate the toxic stagnation over time: improving the flow of Qi; switching a negative feedback cycle back into positive reinforcement.

Chapter 7

The Prevention of Illness in TCM

Part One: Prevention

It is a belief in TCM that a doctor's duty is not simply to prescribe drugs to the sick but to interpret a patient's body: to educate them on what they should and should not do in the pursuit of health — and how they might help themselves in the avoidance of, and in the healing from periods of illness. In TCM, it is the *prevention* of sickness that is so important. History has embedded this philosophy into the Chinese mode of thought as a fundamental contrast to the Western, problem-oriented approach.

TCM doctors build prevention into their medical practice. The head of the family relies on this principle to govern the family, the governor of the city uses this to manage the city, the emperor applies this to maintain the country, and the doctor employs it when 'treating' the body.

When concerned with prevention, we are concerned with what lies within, not without. In TCM, the internal harmony of all the body's parts, as they are governed by the internal Jing Qi Shen and defensive Qi, or Wei Qi, is the key element.

Part Two: Balance is Key

In TCM, recognising the importance of prevention does not mean dismissing the importance of treatment. When discussing a true TCM approach, we should instead observe the right balance *between* prevention and treatment. Treatment is a clear priority for the sick, where illness has already taken hold. However, we may not always recognise when we are sick, while prevention will always support our journey back to health. Unfortunately, we sometimes wait until problems have arisen before we give thought to prevention. Two ancient Chinese proverbs assist us here: 'it is unwise to drill the well when you are already thirsty' and 'it is too late to make weapons if the fighting has already started'.

So, how exactly does TCM implement healthy prevention into a patient's life?

Throughout Chinese history, there have been over 200 Kings and Queens: they all wanted to live long and healthy lives (some even wished to be immortal!). These rulers had countless remedies and potions made for them — many exotic foods and special teas. In the

Qing Dynasty, for example, the emperor drank fresh blood daily, drained from deer, to preserve his energy and vigour. Unfortunately, many did not achieve their goals, and often they instead died young. Regardless of their incredible power and wealth, the health of a King or Queen is as complicated as anyone else's. There is no shortcut, easy fix, or magic potion — we must instead follow the all-important rule: Balance.

In TCM, balance is active in six key ways.

1. A Universal Balance
Our bodies exist in the world alongside many other things — wind, water, sunshine, trees and grass, animals, insects, and so on. We should not distinguish our interior selves from this external world. We and others form a coexisting bond — relying upon one another, influencing each other: sharing space and even, at times, form. Of those things which are not us, TCM follows an ancient dualism: dividing the world into the part above and the part below. The part above our body, the upper part, is called 'Heaven'; the part below, the lower part, is 'Earth'. We are in the middle. Heaven conforms to the sky, sun, air, wind, rains, and snow — elemental forces of scale. The Earth, meanwhile, comprises material sets: water, food, animals, cities, and so on. So, these three parts — heaven, earth, and human together — form the trinity of our living world. This unity of three becomes a tangible world, which is the basic philosophy of the Chinese people and Chinese Traditional Medicine, as discussed in Chapter 2.

This tripartite balance is demonstrated across the cosmos: I–you–him/her, yesterday–today–tomorrow, upper–middle–lower, left–middle–right, length–weight–height, and so on. The body is just one of three parts, and harmony must be kept between it and the other two — heaven and earth. Indeed, following ancient Chinese thought, only when the heaven–human–earth balance is reached can the world tangibly exist. It is in this real world that we thrive, and our lives can be sustained.

The question that naturally follows is, how do we maintain this heaven–human–earth balance? The secret is to follow the rule of nature: namely, the Dao, as discussed in Chapter 2.

Heaven cannot be changed by the body; earth can only be changed with great effort, and then only to minor effect. As such, to maintain the harmony between heaven, body, and earth, the body must be adapted to account for seasonal changes and geographic/material changes. We dress differently in summer than we do in winter — our diets in autumn differ from those in spring. When living beside rivers, we might prepare for a flood, living on mountains, for an avalanche. To thrive, we must adapt our lifestyle to the environment.

In Chinese medical practice, we often advise our patients to adapt their bodies to fit their natural environments: recommending actions that counterbalance the forces of heaven and earth that are acting upon them. During the season of rains, a patient should acclimatise by dressing for rain — eating dry food or hot foods and drinking hot drinks (or even spirits!) that dry out the cold and dampness.

Of course, the concept of cooling, warming, and drying of food is new, and needs a little explanation. TCM does not consider food 'cold' if it just came out of a freezer, or something 'hot' when it's from the oven: these terms refer to their properties. TCM differentiates 'hot', 'cool', 'dry', and 'damp' foods according to the animal or vegetable's relationship to water, land, the seasons, geographical location, and the elements during their growth cycle.

Strong links to water usually confers the 'cool' property to a food, and the opposite is true for that considered 'hot'. For example, rice grows in water, and it is a cooling food, while barley flourishes on dry land as a warming food. Cooking methods also impact the properties of a dish. Boiling or steaming can produce relatively cooling foods, while roasting, baking, or frying contributes to increasing their warmth. Of course, there are some exceptions — but for all foods (as with all things!), origin and treatment result in properties.

2. Balance of Body and Society
Attaining a state of harmony between self and the world is simply a precondition or starting point. Health also requires a balance within the self.

Just as society is positioned between the heaven-human-earth trinity, TCM further considers the human element a composite of three parts: the I (or first person), the you (or second person), and the him/her (or third person). This is the basis of human relations; equality, peace, and humanity derive from a state of balance between these parts, and civilisation is dependent upon this balance. Looking back through history with this traditional Chinese perspective, we should note how imbalance between these parts has led to war, conflict, injury, starvation, and general instability — in turn causing unhealthy bodies, illnesses, and death. Imbalance has even contributed to the collapse of entire civilisations!

In turn, there is also the issue of balance within the body itself. Our bodies comprise many parts, tissues, and organs, which together form a unified organism or whole. All these parts need to be in sustained in harmony to keep the whole in good order, or in health. TCM holds that our bodies are not separate to nature but derive from nature — that the DNA that maps us is the DNA of nature.

Our bodies reflect nature's secrets, and in this respect is like a small universe itself — a universe in microcosm. This 'human universe' can be further divided by this principle to the universe of each organ, and so on, by a fractal logic. All the parts of the body universe or sub-body universes work together to form the unity we call a human being. Each part of this unity relies on the other constituent parts: complementing each other in health, fighting together against sickness, and exchanging energy and form in a kind of conversation or communication.

Mimetically, TCM scholars have likened this system to the organs of state. The King of this small country is the Heart. The Heart is the controlling 'Spirit', or 'Shen' (a kind of force dominating life and soul). The Lung is the premier, or Prime Minister of the body, administrating Qi through breath — channelling the living force. The Spleen is the country's treasurer: tracking the accounts of nutrition, and the supply of nourishment. The Liver is the justice: maintaining harmony through the removal of foreign and corruptive elements. The Kidney is the general: protecting the body from invasions from without and toxins from within.

In TCM, these five organs — the Heart, Lungs, Spleen, Liver, and Kidneys — are considered the innermost. They are the executive powers of the body and reflect the five basic elements of Earth: fire, metal, earth, wood, and water. Other organs, such as the Small Intestine, Large Intestine, Stomach, Gallbladder, and Urinary Bladder, are all subsidiary to the five elemental organs. They all contribute to the complex unity of the human system. If any part of this unity is out of order — too weak or too strong — the harmony of that system is disrupted, which in turn disrupts health and may lead to sickness: just as a tyrannical or absent general, or corrupt or incompetent exchequer, may lead a country to ruin.

Processes of collaboration, combat, and interchange compose the human life cycle, and constitute the living body. All the organs work together as one, and for the one (life) — in turn, the one (life) works for all: a cycle of mutual support that illustrates the essential equilibrium within the human body. In TCM, this internal balance is a precondition to 'health'.

3. Rest Well, Exercise Well
The body is a planet in microcosm. The Earth's waters flow in rivers through to oceans, and in this movement gives the planet life. A body lives through the movement and flow of its parts. To walk, to eat, to study, to sing: we live through acts which are in turn the channelling of flow. TCM calls for moderation in these actions, just as a balanced environment is essential to a stable planet. In other words, exercise accordingly!

Underactivity or overexertion works against the health of the body, and those of different ages should maintain different styles of exercise. Tai Chi works to the pace of elderly bodies where football may not, just as in TCM, we encourage more exercise in the spring and less strenuous activity in the winter, where the body tends towards rest and sleep.

To only rest and do nothing every day is also very unhealthy. Without movement, the Qi becomes easily congested, which in turn will lead to illness. As we say, a flowing river never smells.

4. Balance of Body and Mind

Confucianism, Daoism, and Buddhism inform the Chinese mind on how to live a happy and healthy life. In TCM, the approach to a healthy body draws huge inspiration from them. In *The Yellow Emperor's Canon of Internal Medicine*, it is said that if we live a life simply, without demand (mind), then we will live without illness (body).

In TCM, our Shen, or Mind, can be easily disturbed, and if the Shen is out of balance, the Qi, will also be disturbed: the body's organs and meridians will lapse out of tune, and illness will take hold. Meditation can settle the disturbed Shen, which historically led to the development of exercises such as Qi Gong and Tai Chi: which join exercises of both Shen and Qi. Qi Gong and Tai Chi slow our breathing, dominating our Qi into balance, which in turn leads to the balance of the Shen. Unlike some power exercises like sprinting, boxing, and football, Qi Gong and Tai Chi have more power to heal because they balance the Qi and the Shen.

5. Supplements to Balance

Nowadays, it is common — even fashionable — to take supplements: many people take supplements every day, ostensibly for the prevention of illnesses. Are they right? On this, my opinion is split 50–50.

World food production is industrial in scale and unnatural in method, with farmers relying too heavily on chemical fertilisers and synthetic enhancements. The food grows too fast and contains little in the way of nutrition. I often see patients who have very 'good' diets, but who suffer from anaemia or low vitality regardless. In this sense, perhaps we should *all* supplement our nutrition intake: even in wealthy, Western countries, which supposedly have limitless access to food.

On other hand, some people work through supplements like candy: in large doses, that can be harmful too. I once had an American patient who suffered from bad headaches, and despite all manner of tests could not track this problem to a root cause. Through time spent studying his body and intake, I discovered he took a small bowl of vitamins every day, as he had for many years. He explained that initially he had felt good as a result — filled with energy! However, a few months later, the headaches arose. Following a tongue diagnosis, I recognised stress in his Liver and implemented a range of TCM Liver treatments, while also advising a reduction in supplement use: by which method, he quickly recovered.

Some TCM practitioners position certain foods and drinks as supplements, and in medicinal markets you might find Ling Zi (Ganoderma) mushroom, Ginseng teas, Goji berry snacks, and so on. Some even mix these to prepare 'sex tonics', hair growth tonics and 'long life' tonics! Regardless, my view remains the same: only take them if needed, and then, only in moderation.

A supplement is not innately 'good' or 'bad', but rather is suitable or unsuitable. If a Chinese doctor diagnoses a weakness, then the appropriate tonics should be taken to purposely strengthen the body against illness.

Some of my patients easily catch colds or flu in winter, so I advise them to take those tonics — catered to their bodies and lifestyles — that strengthen their Lungs and Wei Qi. Were they to take too much — or take them indefinitely — their inner balance would again falter! And yet, taken as directed, such supplements can work to restore a body's harmony when environmental conditions might otherwise threaten it with sickness.

6. Maintaining Balance Through Epidemics and Pandemics

Human history is in some respects the history of epidemics and pandemics. They have always been with us. While we have addressed the matter of treatment above (see febrile diseases), TCM also guides our preparation for and the prevention of infectious disease.

As a child, I once experienced an epidemic of meningitis in my home province. The other students and I were stopped outside of the school gates each morning, and before entering we were asked to gargle and then drink a mouthful of herbal tea. This began the day with a ritual that brought our health to the forefront of our minds (and provided the tonic of the tea itself!).[1] During the COVID-19 pandemic, I revived this old technique and urged my patients to gargle and then drink specific teas at the start of every morning.

The TCM tradition also recognises how some natural forces can disrupt environmental harmony — in turn, bringing sickness. The presence of mosquitoes, for instance, can sustain certain infectious diseases in an area: especially malaria. In my hometown, villagers would burn herbs such as Moxa and Qing Hao to smoke out, expel, or kill mosquitos at dusk: the time they emerge in summer. For years, local populations also made nutritious 'cakes' made of Qing Hao — a kind of herb — or drank Qing Hao as tea. In 2015, a Chinese doctor, Professor Tu YouYou, received the Nobel Prize in Medicine for her research proving the effectiveness of Qing Hao in the treatment of malaria.

In this way, we might see how the traditional aspect of TCM can sustain profound insight into the mechanisms

---

[1] Interestingly, TCM techniques also came in handy during this time when working to secure clean water! As a teenage apprentice, when learning to collect and use Chinese herbs under the direction of my masters, we gave a herb called Guan Zhong (Cyrtomium) to rural villagers. We instructed the villagers to plant this herb in and around their wells outside, or water containers inside. As a germicidal plant, the Guan Zhong helped ensure the water was safe to drink — and even sweet!

of environmental harmony — carrying that knowledge forward in the continued pursuit of balance.

By advocating for these six dynamics of balance — and building them into a proactive practice — TCM serves to prevent sickness: not by treating illnesses, but by sustaining health.

Epilogue

In the course of this text, I have endeavoured to explain the reasoning of TCM in the authentic Chinese mode. As has been said, TCM is an ancient practice. Its theories, methods, and treatments formed and evolved far earlier than the scientific method or modern medical ethics. Invariably, one will find aspects of that practice that appear ill suited to a purely scientific, materialistic understanding of the human body, health, illness, and its treatment.

Some aspects of physiology and pathology in the Tradition might be found wanting: incomplete or plain incorrect when approaching it with Western preconceptions. Nevertheless, the same ancient origins that produce this anxiety also provide a grand endorsement: TCM has been playing its role in keeping Chinese people healthy for millennia. Where it *has* been wanting, it has also been modified by the sheer weight of practice and time. So, the Tradition we inherit now is composed of the truest and most *useful* parts — beaten out by the weight of three thousand years and billions of implementations.

From this perspective, Traditional Chinese Medicine is one of the more successful systems of thought in all human history.

The Chinese population comprises almost a quarter of the world's population, and yet today the average lifespan exceeds 75 years. It isn't easy — for *any* medicine — to maintain such health in such a large population: all the while facing the challenges of poverty, wars, and malnutrition. While TCM is far from the only stabilising factor, it is undoubtedly one of the most important factors. Herb treatment, acupuncture, tui na massage, cupping, Qi Gong, Tai Chi, and the many other methods which are used in TCM are still universally applied in China: and now we see them slowly spreading — bringing new meaning to new parts of the world.

The practices of TCM still hold to the old TCM theories: the Yin–Yang dualism of the Dao; the Buddhist notions of Qi and Blood; the traditional folk aspects of the Five Elements, Six Evils, Seven Emotions, and so on. While these philosophies are not all verifiable under the conditions of the scientific method, they nevertheless contain expansive and cohesive internal logics. To the modern Chinese mind, they are not only reasonable but also the constituent parts of Common Sense. In the 40+ years I have practiced TCM, and

through the thousands of patients I have studied, inter-
rogated, and treated, I have myself played a small part
in continuing the process that has carried the Tradition
from the 2nd millennium B.C. through to the present
day: as a Tradition that lives in animation, culture, and
application.

I have been satisfied by the clinical results it has enabled. I would not have devoted myself to it then — or
spent the effort to promote it now — had I not.

In the early chapters of this book, I introduced the
essential aspects of TCM theory and the philosophical
and medical contexts from which it arose. TCM is not
a simple science: and beyond the short introduction
I have provided, I won't try to justify the 'validity' of
TCM with raw data, figures, or meta-studies. I will
leave that aspect of the work to those who come after.

The vast knowledge contained within TCM is not an
easy thing to explain in brief. Confounding this —
many of its formative texts were written in ancient
Chinese — few translations of these texts are available
in the West — and a good deal of detail and meaning
are lost in translation besides. Nevertheless, the bibliography contains a few suggestions of where one *may*
wish to go next to continue the study of the Tradition.

Interestingly, TCM in China is also called 'Zhong Yi'
(or 'Middle Medicine') 中医. I choose to interpret
this as 'the medicine that places things in the middle':

the process of returning a body to its own neutrality. While this is no doubt debatable, it makes keen sense to me. Not too left, nor too right; neither up nor down; neither too hot nor too cold — siding with neither the Yin nor the Yang. The core function of Traditional Chinese Medicine is finding that 'middle' state of balance, alignment, or harmony: between the noun and the verb of it.

Beyond the many details of symptoms and signs, the foundation upon which all TCM treatments are built is an intention to help people restore what is uneven in the body. The prevention of illness follows the same principle. So, balance is everything, and a universal rule: the truth in that common saying, that the best life is one led with everything in moderation. Here, TCM returns to the Daoism from which it first arose; here, TCM is also considered a part of the Dao of life. Beyond the health of the body, it moves out — to the harmony of the family, to the direction of a business, or the governing of a country. For many in China — and perhaps soon, all across the world — TCM is not just a medicine, but a way of life.

Glossary

Auscultation: A diagnostic technique by which the Doctor listens to the patient's heart — typically, though not necessarily, through a stethoscope — noting strength, frequency, and regularity of the pulse.

Ben: As opposed to Biao — translated as 'roots': A metaphor for the core imbalance that predisposes a body to the illnesses that subsequently take hold.

Biao: 'Branches' or 'Leaves' — TCM's metaphor for symptoms — which are regarded as connected, but lesser, issues, as regards the illness (and the imbalance that causes it) proper. Opposed to Ben.

Blood: 'Xue' in Chinese. In Traditional Chinese Medicine, it is said 'Blood is a denser form of Qi; Blood is inseparable from Qi; Qi moves Blood — Blood is the mother of Qi'.

Evil Qi: Forces of imbalance that contribute to sickness or disease. Note that despite the popular translation including the term 'Evil', Evil Qi is not supernatural or mystical.

(The body's) **Five Elements:** The five core internal elements between which internal balance is maintained: (1) Yin/Yang; (2) the body's organs; (3) Jing; (4) Qi; and (5) Shen.

Formulae: The combination of specific herbal remedies in a curative supplement; the classical treatises outlined many thousands of separate formulae.

Fu (Organs): Hollow organs, such as the Stomach and Intestines.

Gao Huang: The deep core of the body, located in the chest, that is difficult to access and treat with DCM.

Jing: Body Essence.

Meridian(s): Paths across the body that are focal points of Qi, through which it flows.

Mirror Tongue: When a patient's tongue does not have any coating. This indicates exhaustion of the Yin and can occur after a long-term sickness.

Olfaction: A diagnostic technique by which the Doctor discovers the extent of — and any disruptions with — the patient's sense of smell.

'Organ'-Qi (e.g., Lung-Qi, Heart-Qi, etc.): Qi that is active through the function and relationships associated with a given organ.

'Organ'-Shen (e.g., Heart-Shen, Liver-Shen, etc.): The Shen (spirit/mind) associated with a given organ.

Palpation: A diagnostic technique in which the Doctor inspects aspects of the body through targeted touch.

Qi: Body Energy.

Qi Gong: A system of exercise and bodily balance techniques, derived from TCM and Daoist practice.

Root Treatment: A TCM treatment that addresses the root cause of an illness: reducing symptoms by tackling the source of those symptoms directly. Usually, this involves rebalancing some aspect of the body that has been disrupted by internal or external Evil Qi.

Shen: Mind (sometimes translated as 'spirit').

Tai Chi/Taijiquan: A system of bodily exercises, derived from Daoism and TCM, which channels the flow of Blood, Jing, and Qi.

Wei Bing: 'Not yet sick'. A body state prior to severe illness, where imbalance has taken hold, though has not yet expressed itself in extreme sickness.

Wei Qi: Defensive Body Energy.

Yang: One half of the Daoist dualism: associated with masculinity, positivity, Heat, summer, light, sun, etc.

Yang-Qi: The Body Energy associated with the body's Yang essence.

Yin: One half of the Daoist dualism: associated with femininity, negativity, Cold, winter, darkness, shade, etc.

Yin-Qi: The Body Energy associated with the body's Yin essence.

Zang (Organs): Solid organs, such as the Heart, Spleen, and Kidney.

Zhen Qi: Vital energy of the body that defends against the Evil Qi — constituted of Qi, Jing, Shen, etc. Zhen Qi is related to Wei Qi.

Zhong Qi: The Middle Qi — the combination of Lung-Qi and Heart-Qi, at the core of a body.

Bibliography

Capra, Fritjof (1975), *The Tao of Physics*, HarperCollins.
    The classic bestseller, exploring the continuity between aspects of ancient Chinese Daoism and contemporary Western theoretical physics.

Li, Shi-zhen (2006), *Compendium of Materia Medica*.
    A complete and comprehensive medical book compiled and written by Li Shi-zhen (1518~1593 A.D.), a medical expert of the Ming Dynasty, over a period of 27 years.

Liu, Yanchi , translated by Fang Tingyu and Chen Laidi (1995), *The Essential Book of Traditional Chinese Medicine: Clinical Practice*, Columbia University Press.
    A modern textbook introduction to TCM in English.

Luo, Guanzhong (1995), *The Romance of the Three Kingdoms*.
    The classic historical text, set in ancient China — a good introduction to the context and background that informed the reification of TCM.

Mi, Huang-Fu (1994), *The Systematic Classic of Acupuncture and Moxibustion*, Blue Poppy Press.
    A formative work in the Tradition — outlining the history, application, logic, and impact of various TCM healing techniques.

Ni, Maoshing (1995), *The Yellow Emperor's Canon of Medicine*, Shambhala Publications Inc.

> The *Huang Di Nei Jing* is traditionally attributed to the Chinese emperor Huangdi, c. 2600 B.C. Modern scholars agree that the text was likely composed closer to c. 300 B.C. by a number of authors. Regardless, the text provides the basis for much of what would become Traditional Chinese Medicine.

Sun, Simiao (2008a), *A Supplement to Prescriptions for Emergencies Worth a Thousand Pieces of Gold*, The Chinese Medicine Database.

Sun, Simiao (2008b), *Prescriptions Worth a Thousand in Gold for Every Emergency*, The Chinese Medicine Database.

> One of two great works of the legendary doctor Sun Simiao — containing thousands of prescriptions and details on acupuncture.

Wang, Lufen (2002), *Diagnostics of Traditional Chinese Medicine*, Shanghai Pujiang Education Press.

> A modern textbook on the Diagnostics of TCM.

Wang, Qin Ren (2000), *The Correction of Traditional Chinese Medicine*, Traditional Chinese Medicine Press.

> Wang took up the Western field of anatomy, dissecting human cadavers and using that knowledge to adjust the understanding of TCM up to that point.

Wen, Jian Min (2003), *Warm Disease Theory* [*Wen Bing Xue*], Redwing Books.

> One of the core canonical works of Traditional Chinese Medicine, featuring examinations of the Heat 'Evil Qi'.

Yang, Shou-Zhong (1998), *The Divine Farmer's Materia Medica: A Translation of the Shen Nong Ben Cao*, Blue Poppy Press.

> One of the three formative texts of TCM. The Tradition attributes the work to the legendary Chinese ruler Shennong, though modern scholars date the

composition to c. 200 B.C.–c. 200 A.D. Sometimes translated as *The Herbal Classic of the Divine Ploughman.*

Zhang, Zhongjing (1995), *Synopsis of Prescriptions of the Golden Chamber with 300 Cases*, New World Press.
Written c. 220 A.D. — one of the core canonical works of Traditional Chinese Medicine — a treatise containing an array of herbal treatments and formulas.

Zhang, Zhongjing (2015), *Discussion of Cold Damage* [*Shang Han Lun*], Singing Dragon Press.
Composed sometime before c. 220 A.D. — one of the canonical works of Traditional Chinese Medicine — containing over 100 herbal treatments and an examination of Cold Syndrome.

Index

64 hexagrams, 31

A

acupuncture, 8–9, 57, 119, 154, 163, 165–166

acupuncture and moxibustion, 15, 17

acupuncture points, 8, 11, 57

acupuncture treatment, 119

auscultation, 129

B

balance, 175, 181–183

Ben, 162, 165

Ben Cao Gang Mu, 18

Biao, 162, 164

blood deficiency, 104, 153–154

blood stagnation, 154–155, 159

body and mind, 3, 36, 181

Body Water, 78, 122, 153–157

Body Water deficiency, 154

Body Water retention, 155

branches and roots, 161–167

Buddhism, 25

C

cause of pain, 154

causes of disease, 73–104

causes of illness, 73

channels, 8

channels and collaterals, 17

Chi, 138

Chinese herbal medicine, 7, 12

Chinese herbal therapies, 7

Chinese medicine, 4, 19

Chinese philosophy, 26, 37

clearing, 170

Cold, 76–77